A short history of breast cancer

W0228150

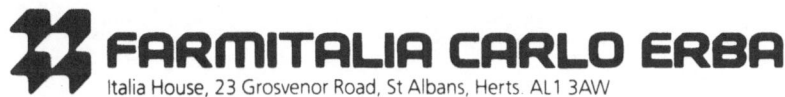

Presented with the
compliments of

FARMITALIA CARLO ERBA

Italia House, 23 Grosvenor Road, St Albans, Herts. AL1 3AW

DANIEL DE MOULIN

Institute of the History of Medicine
Catholic University, Nijmegen, The Netherlands

A short history of breast cancer

KLUWER ACADEMIC PUBLISHERS

DORDRECHT / BOSTON / LONDON

Published by Kluwer Academic Publishers,
P.O. Box 17, 3300 AA Dordrecht, The Netherlands.

Kluwer Academic Publishers incorporates
the publishing programmes of
D. Reidel, Martinus Nijhoff, Dr W. Junk and MTP Press.

Sold and distributed in the U.S.A. and Canada
by Kluwer Academic Publishers,
101 Philip Drive, Norwell, MA 02061, U.S.A.

In all other countries, sold and distributed
by Kluwer Academic Publishers Group,
P.O. Box 322, 3300 AH Dordrecht, The Netherlands.

Second printing (paperback)
ISBN 978-0-7923-0524-8   ISBN 978-94-009-1059-1 (eBook)
DOI 10.1007/978-94-009-1059-1

Cover illustration: silver tetradrachme of the town of Acragas in Sicily.
5th century BC

© 1983 Martinus Nijhoff Publishers
© 1989 by Kluwer Academic Publishers
All Rights Reserved. No part of this publication may be reproduced, stored in a retrieval system,
or transmitted in any form or by any means, mechanical, photocopying, recording or
otherwise, without the prior written permission of the publisher.

Preface

The Third Breast Cancer Working Conference of the Breast Cancer Cooperative Group of the European Organization for Research on Treatment of Cancer, to be held in Amsterdam on April 27–29, 1983, was the principle motive for writing this book. It was felt that a short review of the main pathogenetic conceptions and therapeutic principles which have presented themselves with regard to mammary cancer in the course of Western history, might help to draw a more complete picture of where we stand today. It is not easy to decide which ideas, although discarded, deserve yet to be remembered and which authors from the past may be considered to be truly representative of the scientific climate of their age. Twenty centuries have produced quite a lot of ideas and the number of medical authors who advanced, or rejected, or modified, or revived them, is really uncountable. So the historian has to make a selection and choices are perforce subjective and open to criticism.

In writing this book I tried to consult original sources in the original language as much as possible. These sources were not always strictly medical since I aimed at placing the problem of malignant breast disease — which might serve as a paradigm of cancer in general — in a somewhat wider context. For the history of medicine is not only a history of ideas, but also that of people, of institutions, of society. Studying the sources I realized once again 'the impossibility of dividing the historiography of ideas into a succession of clear-cut stages. More frequently we are dealing with new emphases and tendencies rather than with new creations', as Owsei Temkin, the grand old man of American medical history once wrote.[1]

For want of time I have been forced to make more use than I cared for of secondary sources, for which I relied mainly on the following works.

First and foremost on Jakob Wolff's *Lehre von den Krebskrankheiten von den ältesten Zeiten bis zur Gegenwart*, which appeared between 1907 and 1928. The wealth of information on cancer, stored within these mighty volumes by the diligence of a single author, a practising physician at that, borders on the unbelievable.[2] A more recent work, which stresses the therapy of breast cancer, in the twentieth century in particular, is *Early breast cancer* by Carl M. Mansfield.[3] I had this book at my elbow when working on the present century. C.D. Haagensen's *Diseases of the breast* (1971) was my 'modern' advisor.[4] An extensive paper by the same author entitled *An exhibit of important books, papers and memorabilia illustrating the evolution of the knowledge of cancer* (1933) proved to be a useful bibliography.[5]

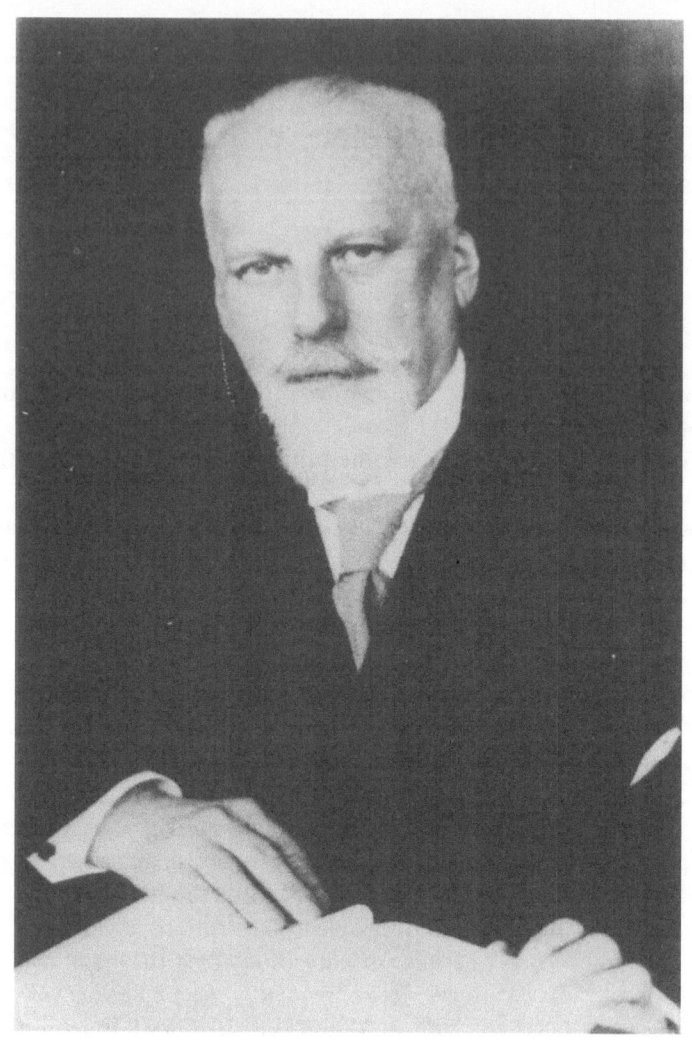

Professor Jakob Wolff (1861–1938),
pre-eminent historiographer of cancer

The help of the following persons is gratefully acknowledged. Marian Poulissen and Mrs Beate van Hasselt, my loyal collaborators and secretaries; Mr. Alexander F. Pleuvry, Macclesfield, Cheshire, United Kingdom, who kindly checked and polished the English; Dr. G.T. Haneveld in Utrecht, a well-known pathologist and medical historian; Mr. E. de Graaff and his staff of the Library of the Nijmegen University Medical School; Mr. A.T.A. Reynen and the staff of the Department of Medical Photography of the Nijmegen University; and, last but not least, my wife.

Contents

List of illustrations

CHAPTER 1

Antiquity

Western medicine has its origins in ancient Greece. It would appear that sometime in the sixth century B.C. the first attempts were being made at explaining the origin and nature of matter and the structure of the universe. Sustained theorising was invented and traditional mythological explanations of natural phenomena no longer satisfied the enquiring mind.

One of the earliest philosophers that Greece produced, was Thales, a merchant living in Miletus on the coast of Asia Minor. He taught that water was the primordial element from which all things are derived. Thales was, moreover, a mathematician and an astronomer, he correctly predicted the solar eclipse of 585 B.C. His fellow townsman and pupil Anaximander postulated that all things were derived from the 'apeiron', an infinite and indeterminate substance. This was a reservoir from which emanated physical contrasts: warm and cold, dry and wet. By their constant competitive inter-action, these elementary contrasts bring about the origin, the being and the decay of things. Anaximander's pupil, Anaximenes, looked upon air as the primary substance that generated all matter. He was the first to recognize that the radiance of the moon is a reflection from the sun. In a different part of the antique world, Sicily, Empedocles of Agrigentum explained the world in terms of four elements: earth, water, air and fire. These are but a few of the natural philosophers who laid the basis of western science, a science which was, to be sure, still highly speculative although based on keen observations. Greek natural philosophy thrived particularly in the Ionian colonies, the coast of Asia Minor, Sicily and southern Italy.

Hippocrates, traditionally considered the founder of rational medicine, was born on the tiny island of Cos, off the coast of Asia Minor, about 460 B.C. At the time of the Trojan war, which took place round about 1200 B.C., the epidemic that hit men and animals alike outside the walls of the besieged city was attributed to the wrath of a god, Apollo, but, in the works of Hippocrates, there is no longer any question of supernatural intervention. The basic philosophy of Hippocratic medicine was the doctrine of the four humours which was to dominate European medical thinking for centuries to come. It was inspired by Empedocles' concept of the four elements. 'The body of man has in itself blood, phlegm, yellow bile and black bile; these make up the nature of his body, and through these he feels pain or enjoys health. Now he enjoys the most perfect health when these elements are duly proportioned to one another in respect of compounding, power and bulk, and when they are perfectly mingled'.[6]

The four cardinal humours in the living body were linked to the four universal elements. Each of the four elements and each of the four humours were endowed with a distinctive pair of elementary qualities, as described by Anaximander. Blood was — like air — moist and hot, yellow bile — like fire — hot and dry, black bile — like earth — hot and dry, phlegm — like water — cold and moist. A perfect state of health depended on a perfect balance of the dynamic qualities incorporated in the humours. There was, of course, little place for anatomy in this essentially humoral concept of health and disease. The practice of Hippocratic medicine was based on careful observation of the patient and his surroundings. One of his characteristic short case-histories bears on breast cancer: 'A woman of Abdera had a carcinoma of the breast and there was a bloody discharge from the nipple. When the discharge was brought to a stand-still she died'.[7]

Hippocrates was aware of 'karkinos' or 'karkinoma' — he used these synonymously — of the nose, the uterus, the breasts and the neck. He associated the origin of breast cancer with the cessation of menstruation. Suppression of menstrual discharge would lead to engorgement of the breast and the appearance of nodules which would become increasingly indurated and ultimately degenerate into 'hidden' cancer. Hippocrates probably used the term 'hidden' cancer to mean tumours which had not yet penetrated the skin. As we will have occasion to remark later in this chapter, there was some confusion as to the exact meaning of this expression. The development of cancer was associated with a bitter taste in the mouth, loss of appetite, disturbed intelligence, dry eyes and nostrils, and loss of smell. Pains radiated from the breast to collar bone and scapula and the patient complained of thirst. The breast was exsiccated and the entire body emaciated.[8] Hippocrates was extremely reserved as to the efficacy of medical treatment: 'It is better to give no treatment in cases of hidden cancer; treatment causes speedy death, but to omit treatment is to prolong life'.[9] This implies that only ulcerated cancer should be treated by operation, possibly as attempted palliation although this concept does not clearly occur in ancient oncology. It was by no means unethical at the time, to send patients away to whom medicine had nothing to offer. Votive offerings representing breasts, excavated at sites where formerly sanctuaries of the Greek healing god Asklepios stood, suggest that breast ailments were amongst those diseases for which supernatural help was occasionally called in (Fig. 2). Hippocrates owes his fame to the celebrated *Corpus Hippocraticum*, a collection of about sixty medical treatises dating from the fifth and fourth century B.C. The *Corpus* was compiled about 300 B.C. in Alexandria on the Nile. It is obvious, however, that the collection consists of books of different authors from different schools.

Alexandria was founded by Alexander the Great in 332 B.C., on the site indicated by Homer, when that venerable poet appeared to him in a dream. Under the royal house of the Ptolemies that ruled Egypt after the early death of the Macedonian conquerer, Alexandria rapidly expanded into a world center of Hellenist science. In its flourishing period, the third and second centuries B.C., no less than 14,000 students studied there at the same time under the guidance of competent teachers. The mathematician Euclides, the astronomers Hipparchus and Hero, the anatomists Herophilus and Erisistratus and — very much later — the physician Galen, were directly or indirectly connected with the Alexandrian school. This 'school' contained botanical

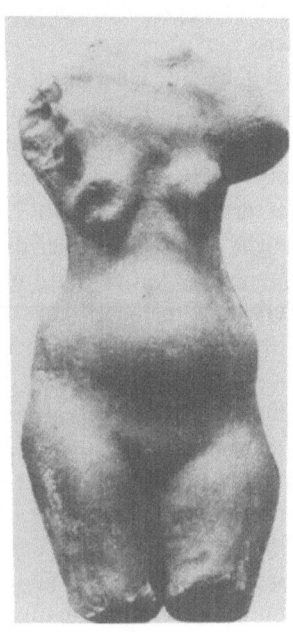

Fig. 2.   Greek votive offering, representing a woman with a breast tumor.

and zoological gardens, an observatory, anatomical theatres and libraries. At one time, these libraries possessed more than 700,000 scrolls, the vastest collection of books that ever existed in antiquity.

Anatomy flourished, giving rise to a form of surgery that distinguished itself from Hippocratic surgery by more sophisticated techniques and tools. The introduction of the vascular ligature in particular led to the expansion of operative surgery.[10]

Between round about 300 and 100 B.C. there were many fine surgeons in Alexandria. Outstanding amongst them was Praxagoras of Cos (fourth century B.C.), who advocated laparotomy in some cases of intestinal obstruction, with incision of the rectum and enterorrhaphy after removal of the obstructing bowel contents.[11] On cancer we find criteria by which it might be possible to distinguish malignant growths.[12]

It is to be regretted that only small parts of the original works of the Alexandrian anatomists and surgeons have survived. Innumerable book scrolls were irretrievably lost in fires that took place during the siege of the city by Julius Caesar in 47 B.C. and again during religious quarrels a few centuries later. Whatever survived these calamities, was dispersed in the winds after the conquest of Alexandria by the Arabs in 642 A.D. The Alexandrian medical legacy consists mainly of short abstracts and isolated fragments of lost works that have been incorporated into compilations composed by several Greek-Byzantine authors living in the fourth to seventh centuries. We will refer in the following to two of them, Aetius of Amida, a Byzantine court-physician of the sixth century, and Paul of Aegina, who presumedly lived in Alexandria shortly before its capture. A great deal of Alexandrian medical lore is further incorporated in the works of Celsus and Galen.

The Roman Aulus Cornelius Celsus lived in the first century A.D. in Gallia Narbonensis, nowadays called Provence. This is about all that we know of him. His *De Medicina*, written in elegant Latin, gives an excellent survey of contemporary medicine, which was essentially Greek. The well-known verse by Horace: 'Graecia capta ferum victorem cepit et artes intulit agresti Latio' (Conquered Greece won over her brute victor and brought the arts to uncivilized Italy) certainly applied to medicine. Celsus' work was not widely known until it appeared in print in Florence in 1478. It was one of the very first medical books to be laid in the press, it was printed even before the works of Hippocrates and Galen.

It is in Celsus' treatise that we find, for the first time, a clinical description of cancer: 'This disease occurs mostly in the upper parts of the body, in the region of the face, nose, ears, lips, and in the breasts of women, but it may also arise in an ulceration, or in the spleen. Around the spot is felt a sort of pricking; there is a fixed, irregular swelling, sometimes there is also numbness. Around it are dilated tortuous veins, pallid or livid in hue; sometimes in certain cases they are even hidden from view; and in some the part is painful to the touch, in others there is no feeling. And at times the part becomes harder or softer than natural, yet without ulcerating; and sometimes ulceration supervenes on all the above signs. The ulceration at times has no special characteristic; at times it resembles what the Greeks call condylomata, both in a sort of roughness and in size; its colour is either red or like that of lentils'.[13] Celsus was also the first to draft a clinical classification. He distinguished four stages: 'cacoethes' ('malignancy'; Celsus did not explain the term further), carcinoma without ulcer, ulcerated cancer, and, lastly, originating from the ulcer 'thymium', a growth that resembled the flowers of thyme and bled easily. He rejected any treatment of the latter three stages, be it by caustic medicaments, the cautery or the scalpel. Any aggressive measure would only irritate the process and, even if the surgeon succeeded in healing the wound of the operation, the disease would inevitably recur. Successful treatment, he declared, would only be possible in the first stage. It was, however, far from easy to distinguish a 'cacoethes' that would respond favourably to treatment from a cancer that would not.

Celsus did not go into the details of surgical treatment. For a full description of the way the operation was performed early in the Christian era, we should turn to Aetius, one of the Byzantine compilators. In his chapters on breast cancer he related what Archigenes and Leonides, a physician and a surgeon of the Alexandrian school which flourished towards the end of the first century, had written on the subject.[14] Both authors, who enjoyed a great reputation in their day, distinguished between cancers with and without ulcers. The non-ulcerated form appears as a bulky swelling, hard on the touch and uneven, 'fierce like a wild animal', sending its roots, surrounded by varicose veins, inwards over a great distance. Its colour is grey to red. It causes stinging pains, radiating sometimes even to the clavicula and scapula. The pain is not brought on by the morbid condition as such, but by the heaviness of the retracted nipple. Malignant inflammations and glands are frequently found in the axillae. Ulcerated cancers are steadily corroding. They cannot be halted and discharge matter that is more poisonous than any poison of the wild animals and gives off a horrible smell. Patients with cancer in the breasts are to be regarded as lost, just like those with similar affections of the head, shoulders, arm-pits and groins. Such swellings cannot be completely removed and are liable to profuse haemorrhages. Only tumours in the summit of the breast which do not occupy more than half of that structure are suitable for surgical treatment. When the whole breast is hardened and the indurated tumour is fixed to the thorax, the surgeon should abstain from operating.

Before resorting to treatment of any malignant process, a general detoxification of the body should be undertaken by purging and by administering theriac (a universal antidote composed of numerous odd ingredients and widely used until well into the nineteenth century) and other draughts, or warm blood of a goose or a duck. Crawfish boiled in ass's milk was also considered to have cleansing effects.[15]

Crawfish has been a popular cancer remedy for many centuries. Its use proceeds from the ancient doctrine of signatures, which still occurs in folk medicine. It is based on the belief that a feature in the appearance or qualities of a natural object or even its name is indicative of its therapeutic utility: 'cancer', the crab, cures 'cancer', the tumour. Unlike Galen and most other authors from antiquity, Archigenes and Leonides did not connect the name of the disease with the swollen veins that are suggestive of the limbs of a crab, but with the characteristic of that crustacean to retain tenaciously whatever it seized in its pincers. The crab was not yet a symbol of cancer as it is today. Since fish was — and still is — a staple food in Mediterranean countries, it is not rare to find that animal portrayed on antique Greek coins[16] (Fig. 3).

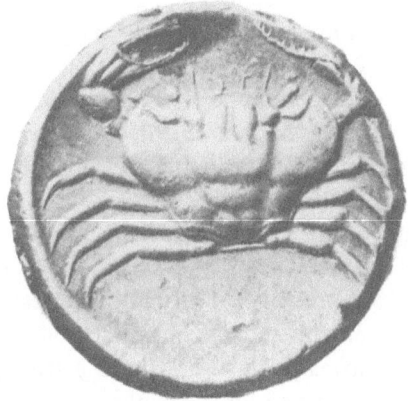

Fig. 3.   Silver tetradrachme of the town of Acragas.

Operative treatment of breast cancer was described by Leonides in the following words (for original text see Fig. 4):

I make the patient lie on her back. Then I make an incision into the sound part of the breast above the cancer and I apply cauteries until an eschar is produced that stops the bleeding. I then make another incision and cut into the deep of the breast

5

Cancri chirurgia, Leonidæ. **Cap. XLV.**

Ego quidem in cācris in pectore obortis chirurgia uti
soleo,quę sic fit.Aegram supinam decumbere facio.
Deinde supra cancrum partem mammæ sanam inci
do,& incisam cauterijs inuro,donec crusta inducta
sanguinis eruptio sistatur.Mox iterum incido &
profundum mammæ disseco,ac rursus partes incisas
uro,sæpeq; idem repeto,& secans,& sistendi sangui
nis gratia inurens.Ita enim sanguinis eruptionis periculum euitatur:post amputationem uerò integrè
peractam,rursus partes omnes ad resiccationē usq;
inuro:et primæ quidē inustiones sistendi sanguinis
gratia fiunt.Postremæ uerò ad omnes morbi reli-
quias abolendas.Sæpe uerò etiam citra inustionem
opus perfeci,ubi induratus tumor cancri generatio-
nem minās in mamma fuit:tali enim affectioni amputatio usq; ad sanam partem sufficit,quum nullum
hic periculum eruptionis sanguinis immineat.

Fig. 4.   Operative treatment of breast cancer, as described by Leonides in the first century AD.

and again sear the severed parts. This I repeat often, alternately cutting and burning
in order to arrest the bleeding. For in this way the danger of haemorrhage is
avoided. When the amputation is completed, I burn once again all parts until they
are dry. The first cauterisations are made for the purpose of arresting haemorrhage.
The rest however with the intention of eradicating all remnants of the disease.
Often, however, I even completed the task without resorting to the cautery, namely
in such cases where an indurated tumour threatened to turn into a cancer in the
breast. For in such a case an amputation up to the sound part suffices since here
no danger of haemorrhage is threatening.[17]

Leonides apparently adapted the extension of the operation to the clinical stage.
Instructions for the after-treatment consisting of different poultices as well as a diet
in which cold beverages and food which is difficult to digest are proscribed, conclude
this earliest known treatise on the surgery of breast cancer. It was not this treatise,
however, that became the starting-point of a rational active approach to the problem
of mammary cancer. This was reserved for the works of Galen.

The Greek Galen, born in Pergamum on the Mediterranean coast of Asia Minor
round about 130 A.D., is one of the great figures in the history of medicine (Fig. 5).
He had studied in Alexandria for some time before settling in Rome, where he lived
and practised for the rest of his life and gained great distinction. He was a keen student
of anatomy and experimental physiology. His literary legacy consists of nearly a
hundred books on many aspects of medicine. They are the result of an ambitious
effort to describe and summarize the entire medical knowledge of his time. His
pathology was based on humoralism. Taking up its principles, as they had been

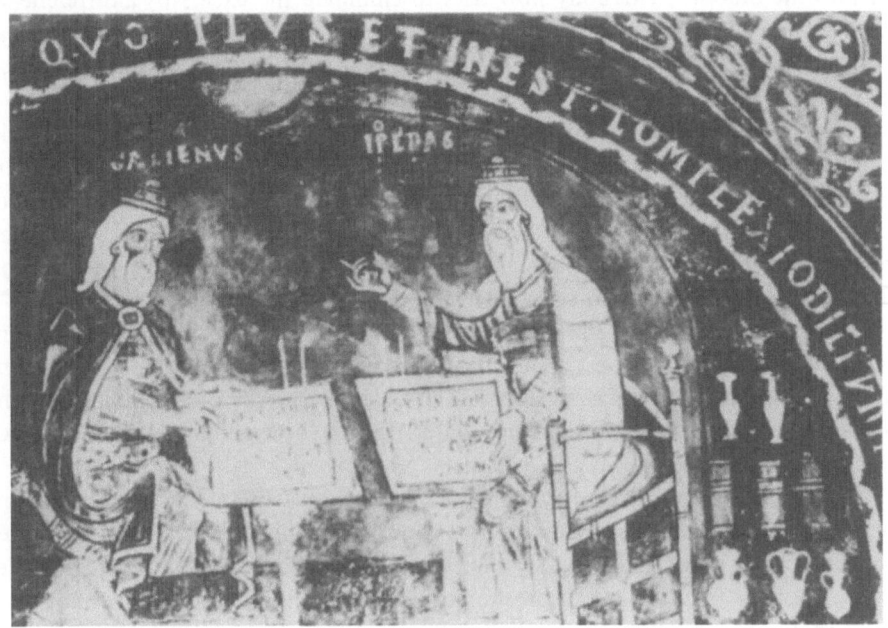

Fig. 5.   Galen and Hippocrates.

explained by Hippocrates, Galen extended this theory to a doctrine which was to dominate medicine for many centuries. Galen's humoralistic views find a clear expression in his discussions of malignant growth.

By preternatural growth ('para physin onkos') Galen understood any form of unnatural increase of mass in the body: malignant and benign tumours, inflammations, aneurysms, skin diseases, ulcers, oedema.[18] In many instances its cause was a localized accumulation of one of the humours. A collection of blood, for instance, would give rise to an inflammation, a congestion of yellow bile to erysipelas, a retention of phlegm to oedema.[19]

Accumulation of thick and slow humour would produce scirrhi. A scirrhus was defined by Galen as a hard and heavy tumour, immovable and insensible. It seems that he did not include scirrhus among the malignancies, in contrast to carcinoma, which he described as a malignant, very hard tumour, whether or not showing ulceration.[20] The latter would be caused by a congestion of black bile. Should this black bile be of a sharp nature, ulcerations would occur.[21]

Black bile, endowed with the elementary qualities of cold and dryness, was to play a paramount part in medical thinking. It looks like dregs and originates in the liver as a by-product of the formation of blood. From the liver it is transported to the spleen where it is absorbed. Together with the veins, the uterus, the skin and the mucous membranes, the spleen was regarded as having cleansing properties. In case the liver produces too great quantities of black bile, or in case the spleen is in a weakened condition, not all black bile can be resorbed in the spleen and a certain amount runs

7

over into the blood.[22] The body now tries to eliminate the excess by a different way and this can lead to haemorrhoids and varicose veins. In women, menstruation means a monthly purification of the entire system; when it fails to come, all sorts of troubles may ensue.[23]

An excess of black bile renders the blood black and thick. The thicker and blacker the blood, the more malignant the afflictions that it generates. Harmful constituents of the blood may precipitate either in the skin, or in some deeper parts of the body. In the first case chronic ulcers and leprosy ensue, in the second case carcinoma. Accumulation of black bile may take place everywhere in the body, more in particular, however, in the breasts of women who no longer menstruate.[24]

Mammary cancer makes itself known by a swelling and by distended veins, reminiscent of the feet of a crab.[25] An inflammatory swelling is tender, a scirrhus is not painful on palpation. This was more or less all Galen had to say of the clinical features. Nowhere did he mention metastasis nor did he describe how patients come to die from the disease.

Therapy of breast cancer may either be conservative or operative, Galen wrote. Since inspissated black bile is the ultimate cause, it stands to reason to try to prevent or at least check its production. To this end the patients should be purged and bled. In women under fifty menstruation should be restarted, if it had stopped: hot baths, walks, frictions and other external therapies would serve the purpose. Ever since Hippocrates the ancient doctors had a long list of emmenagogues at their disposal.[26] A proper nutrition should be observed. The diet of these patients must consist of sieved barley infusion and milk-whey in particular, malva, atriplex (a plant of the goosefoot family) and pumpkin are recommended as vegetables. With regard to fish, he allows only those kinds living between the rocks. Except for water-fowl, there is no restriction as to birds.[27]

Local treatment consists of the application of the juice of 'strychnos' (nightshade) or of 'pompholyx' (impure oxide of zinc) that is also indicated in ulcerated cases. The ulcer base should be cleansed by ablutions with emollient agents. In hidden cases 'chalcites' (a copper mineral, probably copper-vitriol) is recommended. Chalcites was included among other copper minerals, lime arsenic and sandrak among the caustics: medicaments with an effect comparable to that of fire.[28] They were in use until well into the nineteenth century.

With the methods just described, Galen claimed to have been successful more than once in early cases, particularly when the atrabiliary humour was not too thick.[25] This statement encouraged many surgeons in the following centuries to adopt a conservative attitude. If, however, the tumour had grown into a substantial mass, nothing but surgery could offer any hope of a cure.

There was apparently some discussion at the time on the correct indication or even on the basic virtue of an operative approach of cancer of the breast. Many physicians held that the operation should be reserved for desperate cases as when the ulcerating tumour inflicts such pain that the patient, at her wits' end, would even be capable of operating upon herself. Others felt that no indication whatsoever could possibly exist for surgical treatment.[29] Some give centuries earlier, Hippocrates had advised against operative treatment in hidden cancers, as we have noted before. Galen quite agreed with the venerable physician of Cos, provided that 'hidden' cancer meant cancer occurring within the body: in the mouth or in the uterus or at the seat (the anus?). It would have been different, if Hippocrates by his term 'occult cancer' had wanted to indicate that no ulceration had as yet set in, an interpretation adhered to by many. For when the tumour is situated on the surface of the body, Galen argued, it might be possible to eradicate it roots and all. In Galen's terminology, roots were not protrusions of the tumour but the dilated veins, filled with morbid black matter.[29] Operative treatment should aim at excision of the preternatural tumour at the boundary between diseased and healthy parts. The surgeon must be well aware, however, of the danger of profuse haemorrhage from large blood vessels. Should he arrest the bleeding by ligating the cut vessels, there would be a definite risk of the surrounding healthy parts being affected by the noxious humour locked up in the tied blood vessels. The use of cautery in destroying the main 'roots' on the other hand entails the hazard that the burning will be more extensive than is strictly necessary.[25]

When, however, the surgeon dares to take the risk, he is to begin with purgings to evacuate the atrabiliary humour. After having cut away the whole diseased part, he must allow the blood to flow freely for a while. Instead of arresting the haemorrhage right away, he should squeeze out the vessels to expel the thick part of the blood.[30] Some surgeons used red-hot knives which enabled them to cut and to burn at the same time.

In Galen's impressive work, ancient medicine had reached its highest point of culminated knowledge. Since it seemed that Galen had laid down in these pages all that could possibly be said on medicine, he attained an authority that remained unchallenged until well into the sixteenth century. His views on cancer continued to be decisive for an even longer time.

After Galen, ancient medicine did not produce any other original contributions. Typical of late antiquity were medical compendia of a practical nature, and collections of recipes. Recipe collections may also be met with in much earlier times. Well known was *Compositiones medicamentorum*, compiled by Scribonius Largus, a contemporary of Celsus, who practised in Rome in the first century A.D. We borrow one recipe from his collection which has a bearing on our subject: 'The following composite medicament cleanses marvellously, also when cancer threatens, yet it is mild. Auripigment (as arsenic is being called by the Greeks): 6 drachms. Scale of copper: 3 drachms. Juice of the springcucumber: 1 drachm. Ashes of burnt paper: 3 drachms'.[31] Arsenic, which we will meet repeatedly in the chapters to come, thus appears to have been in use in the treatment of cancer, as early as the beginning of the Christian era. Galen too, used arsenic as we have seen.

Scribonius' contemporary, the Latin poet Ovid, described in his *Metamorphoses* how the Athenian girl Aglauros was petrified from sheer envy of her sister, who had attracted the attention of Mercury, the good-looking herald and messenger of the gods: 'And just like cancer, that irremediable ailment, is wont to eat away far and wide, joining the parts that are still unaffected to those already in corruption, in such a manner the cold of death penetrated into her body and closed off all ways of the vital breath'.[32] Cancer had become paradigmatic of a living process of a particularly evil nature.

9

CHAPTER 2

The Middle Ages

In the history of Europe, the period between the political downfall of the Western Roman Empire in 576 and the discovery of America in 1492 is usually called the Middle Ages. The concept of 'ages lying in between' arose in the Renaissance, which strove to imitate a strongly idealized antiquity.

The downfall of the Western Roman Empire did not, for some time, bring about very radical changes in daily life in Western − and Southern − Europe. Until the end of the sixth century, the traditional economic and cultural contacts with the countries in the Near East remained undisturbed. After the advancing Arabs had occupied the east, south and west coasts of the Mediterranean in the seventh century, trade relations between Western Europe and the Near East virtually came to an end. Soon the Danes started to raid the north coasts of the old continent and the ancient trade-routes to Eastern Europe were being blocked by invading Huns and Hungarians. Consequently, Western Europe became a closed area in which, during the ninth to eleventh centuries, foreign trade largely came to a standstill. The result was, among other things, a relapse to a more primitive form of economy, in which everything that is produced by the soil or by human hands is used for home consumption.[33]

Obviously, there was little or no use for science in such rather primitive, isolated communities, which suffered, moreover, from many internal wars. Only in the Church there were men who were able to read and to write. Whatever theological, scientific and medical writings had been preserved were kept almost exclusively in monastic libraries, where they were read, copied, digested and collected into anthologies. Original contributions to scientific medicine were not made during these two centuries.

Figure 6 shows a page of a manuscript representative of ninth century medical writing.[34] This codex was written in the famous abbey of Reichenau on the island of the same name in Lake Constance. The text is anonymous and bears no title, but the present writer was able to identify it as a Latin translation of the last chapters of a pseudo-Galenic treatise called *Introductio sive medicus*. In bad Latin it says on this page, among other things: 'Cancrum fit in multa loca corporis, maxime in mamillis et inciditur ubicumque fuerit et igni circumdatur et simul et statim incidere oportet' (Cancer occurs in many parts of the body, mostly in the breasts and it is incised wherever it may be and it is on all sides surrounded with fire applied by the cautery and one should incise it as soon as it is recognized and henceforth.) The simultaneous use of the knife and the cautery reminds us of Leonides and these lines may well be

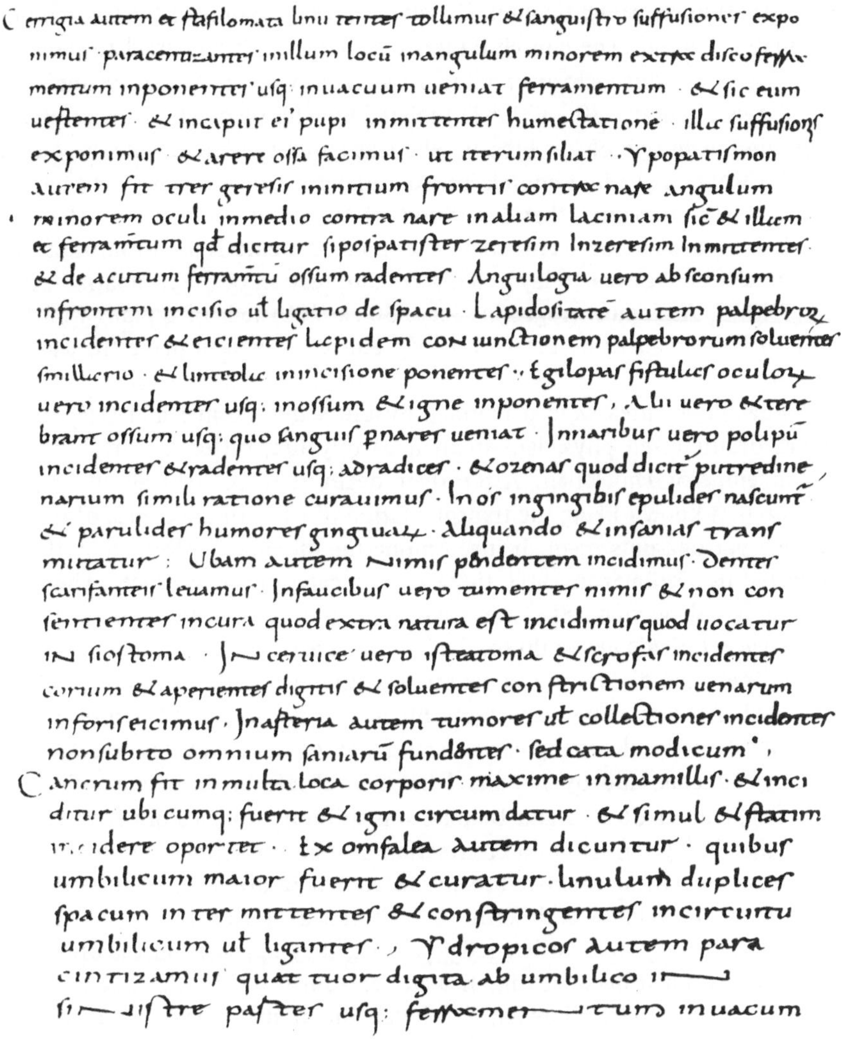

Fig. 6. A medical text from the ninth century.

a poor summary of his mastectomy technique. On the basis of this scanty information no physician or surgeon would ever have been able to recognize and treat cancer. No other treatise of the time, however, gives any more details. Manuscripts like this one can at best have served as a general introduction to medicine or may perhaps have served as encyclopaedic information for non-medical readers. However, such information cannot have been much in demand because of the prevailing illiteracy. Medicine, as it was practised mainly by monks, consisted of a primitive sort of popular medicine. Surgery was of a most elementary kind, practised not by the clergy but by empirics.

Whenever human medicine is deficient, man is inclined to look for help and consolation from supernatural powers. In antiquity it was the healing god Asklepios whose intervention was sought, and in Christian times the Saints of the Church or even God the Father himself. The church-fathers encouraged this and tried to substantiate the superiority of divine help over human medicine with numerous examples. Thus Gregory of Nyssa (about 330–400 A.D.) related how his own sister had suffered from a horrible tumour in one of her breasts. She was cured in a miraculous way after she had passed a whole night in a church, prostrated before the altar and had smeared the stricken part with the mud that her flood of tears had produced on the floor.[35] The spending of a night in a church in the hope of a cure is a custom that prevails in the Oriental Church even today as a direct continuation of the incubation practised in the temples of Asklepios. Augustine (ca. 330-ca. 400) tells of a pious woman who was cured of breast cancer by having a newly converted person make the sign of the cross over it.[36]

Many miraculous cures were performed by the Saints Cosmas and Damian. These holy twins, disinterested physicians in their earthly life, suffered martyrdom under the Roman emperor Diocletian. After their death they brought about wonderous healings, the best-known being the transplantation of a leg. In the course of time, they have become patron-saints of medicine. Among the 48 cures performed by them that were collected by Deubner in 1907, there are two cases of breast cancer. The first one concerned a Jewish woman. She was advised by the holy brothers to eat pork, but since her religion forbade her to do so, she laid the meat that was handed out to her on her bosom. There the disease was transferred to the meat, and the woman was cured and converted. An interesting aspect of this legend is the part played by the pork: laying raw meat on an ulcerating cancer was a way of treatment that was occasionaly practised by surgeons and by popular healers until late in the nineteenth century. The second patient of Cosmas and Damian was suffering from a stone-hard tumour in the breast, that had given rise to a contraction around the nipple. Her doctor advised her to have an operation when it became clear that resolvent medicines were of no avail. The woman declined and went to a church dedicated to the two saints for consolation. When they noticed her religious zeal, they appeared in the dream of one of the doctors who had been treating her and explained to him the way in which he should do the mastectomy, showing the details on an anatomical model which they had brought along. But when next day the doctor went into the church with his instruments in order to act according to his instructions, he was amazed to find that the woman had already been operated upon. On further consideration the saints had apparently thought it better to do the operation themselves, leaving only the after-treatment to their worldly colleague.[37] It is striking that the saints, just like Asklepios before them, had made use of methods that were practised in human medicine to achieve their goal.

Saint Agatha, a martyr in Sicily in the middle of the third century whose two breasts were cut off, has come to be regarded as a patron-saint for breast disease (Fig. 7).

From the eleventh century there was an increase in sea traffic. Renewed commercial contacts with countries outside the continent greatly improved the general level of prosperity and with this improval went a revival of arts and sciences, as testified by the rise of Gothic style, Gregorian music and the creation of magnificent manuscripts

12

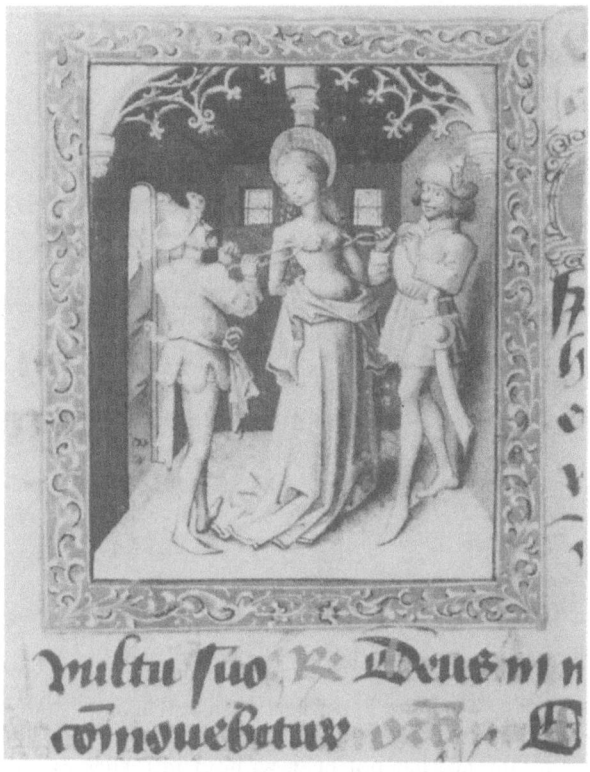

Fig. 7. St. Agatha.

including quite a few on medicine. Surgery, too, was developing, first in Italy but before long also in France. The flourishing of surgery in the later Middle Ages was connected with the rise of universities in Northern Italy in the twelfth and thirteenth centuries and with the introduction of Arabian medical literature in Europe. The Arabs had come to know antique Greek science when they were expanding their empire in the Near East in the seventh century. They took it, translated into Arabic, with them to Spain where they established important centres of culture and science. There, these writings were once more translated, now into Latin, which made them accessible to the western world. By this detour, antique science once again became known in Europe.

Original contributions of Arabic authors, in Latin translation, too, penetrated the West: the celebrated *Canon* of Avicenna, for instance, which until well into the seventeenth century had the reputation of being second only to Galen's work. What Avicenna had to say on breast cancer, though, is of little interest.

More important for our theme are the chapters on surgery from the *Altasrif* of Abulcasis (Abul-Qasim, 936–1013) which, even though it was highly inspired by the Byzantine compilator Paul of Aegina, contains numerous observations of his own. He liked to work, as he elaborately explained, with the cautery and with caustic

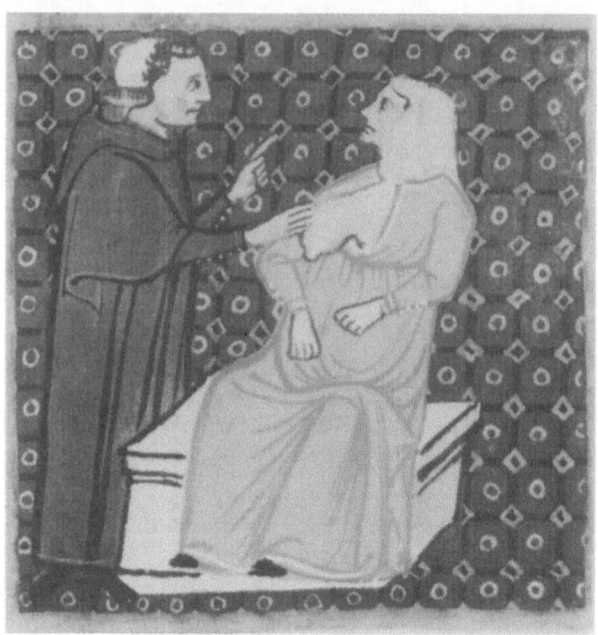

Fig. 8.   Teodorico Borgognoni: examination of the breast.

medicines and this preference has not been without influence on operative surgery in Europe. Abulcasis was already frequently cited in the first important surgical works that appeared in Europe. In his treatment of breast cancer he followed Paul of Aegina who, in his turn, based his oncological chapters on Galen. As a personal comment he gloomily added: 'I for one never could cure one single case, nor do I know anybody else who succeeded in doing so':[38]

In the splendid works of the Italian Renaissance surgeons of the later Middle Ages such as Bruno da Longoburgo (1252), Guglielmo da Saliceto (1258) and Teodorico Borgognoni (1275), the subject of mammary carcinoma is treated entirely from a Galenic point of view (Fig. 8). Black bile being the proximate cause, it is obvious that the attempt should be made to remove this harmful tumour by rigorous purging and by phlebotomy and to limit its production as much as possible by appropriate dietary measures. Patients should be dissuaded from taking salt, sharp, sweet or sour food, garlic, vegetables, cheese and full and sweet wine, stated Guglielmo. He furthermore advised guarding the patient from excitement and not allowing any heavy work. He gave a number of recipes of compounds to be used for local treatment: salves containing Armenian bolus, leadwhite, terra sigillata, rose-powder, myrtle-leaf powder. For a stronger effect deadly nightshade, juice of wall-pepper, of purslane, and of lettuce should be added, as well as rose-water and oil of violets.[39]

None of the three Italians believed in operating. Excision only serves the purpose, Guglielmo wrote, in imitation of Galen, when it is feasible to remove the entire growth with all its roots — apparently conceived as inwards protusions. Bruno was the only

14

one to give any details of the operation. It consisted of lifting the breast with a hook and excising it from its surroundings. The severed veins should be allowed to empty – to evacuate the melancholic blood in accordance with Galen's advice – and the wound surface be seared with red-hot cautery. In case the patient refused an operation or was too weak to stand it, Bruno believed treatment with caustics was indicated.[40] Teodorico relied heavily on Galen in his short chapter on cancer, but added a description of how untreated patients come to an end. The morbid process spreads over the entire chest and may give rise to a lethal haemorrhage or to a putrefying sore with fevers that, in the end, will also lead to death.[41]

Guglielmo's book was the first to contain chapters on surgical anatomy. Nothing was said, however, relating to the anatomy of the breasts.

More on surgical anatomy can be found in the *Chirurgie* of Henri de Mondeville (1260?–1320), the most important representative of the older French surgeons. He practised in Montpellier and in Paris as well as in the army as a private surgeon to Philip-the-Handsome. What he had to say on breasts does not exactly testify to a sound knowledge of anatomy, but is not entirely devoid of charm: 'The reasons why the breasts of women are on the chest, whereas other animals more often have them elsewhere, are of three kinds. First, the chest is a noble, notable and chaste place and thus they can be decently shown. Secondly, warmed by the heart, they return their warmth to it so that this organ strengthens itself. The third reason applies only to big breasts which, by covering the chest, warm, cover and strengthen the stomach'.[42] Just like his contemporaries, Henri de Mondeville had little opportunity to acquaint himself with anatomy by dissecting dead bodies. He devoted comprehensive treatises to the aetiology, the symptomatology and the therapy of cancer.[43] Its cause may be either internal or external. The internal cause is combusted and putrified melancholy, either melancholy which normally occurs in the body as black bile, or melancholy which arises from previous combustion of other body humours and which is, after having been burnt for a second time, potentially more malignant than natural black bile. The notion that black bile may not only be generated in a 'natural' way in the liver, but can also present itself as a waste product of blood, yellow bile or phlegm, does not seem to occur in the treatises of ancient authors, insofar as these have been preserved.

The first, natural species may give rise to the formation of a hard induration, named 'sklerosis' by Henri de Mondeville. This condition is to be distinguished from real cancer, which originates from non-natural, twice-combusted black bile. External causes may be wounds or ulcers that have been treated inexpertedly, or contusions. The cancer sore is round, having thick, raised and inverted margins. It shows cavities, its base is hard and lumpy, livid or blue. It spreads a most offensive fetor defying any description: experienced surgeons can diagnose the disease at the mere smell without even having seen it. Treatment once again is tripartite: diet, purging and possibly operation. Operation consists, just as with Galen, of excision, emptying of the cut veins and cautery. Surgical treatment only makes sense, however, when the growth can be totally eradicated all at once. If one abstains from operating and wishes to use caustic agents instead, sublimated arsenic should be resorted to since all practitioners agree that there is no better cauterant. More often than not, treatment can be merely palliative. The surgeon should only proceed to any sort of treatment at the urgent request of the patient and after having pocketed a substantial fee. Apparently, Henri feared that, after the death of the patient, the surgeon might ask for his money in vain.

Henri concluded his first chapter on breast cancer with some very interesting reflections on quack remedies that may be hung around the neck of the patient. It is a fact, he stated, that a number of such remedies can sometimes effect unbelievable cures in desperate cases in which medical aid has been of no avail. Constantinus Africanus (Constantine the African, ca. 1020–ca. 1087), a monk in Montecassino, who by his unflagging industry in translating medical works played an important part in the introduction of Arab science in the Latin West, had already called attention to the force of imagination in his book *De incantationibus et conjurationibus, sortilegiis, maleficiis, medicinis suspensis ad collum et ad alias partes corporis* (On incantations and conjurations, sortileges, charms, medicines hung around the neck and on other parts of the body). Henri de Mondeville recalled the opinion of this mediaeval authority, who was apparently not lacking in psychosomatic understanding: if one succeeds in stimulating the healing force of the soul by incantations and that sort of thing and meanwhile continues to treat the body with appropriate medicines, cure will be effected all the sooner.

Henri de Mondeville's book was less widely read and therefore exerted less influence on the history of surgery than that by his famous pupil Guy de Chauliac (1300–?), court-physician to the popes Clemens VI and Innocentius VI, residing in Avignon. Guy left, among other things, a moving description of the plague-epidemic that afflicted Avignon in 1348. He was on good terms with Francesco Petrarca who lived for some time in Avignon, although the latter thoroughly disliked physicians in general since they had not been able to prevent his beloved Laura from dying of plague.

Guy's main work was his *Grande Chirurgie*, however. It was written in 1363 and at least 34 mediaeval manuscripts survive, written in Latin, French and other languages. From the fifteenth until the seventeenth century some 69 printed editions appeared in a wide diversity of languages. Nothing special on the subject of breast cancer, however, can be found in this celebrated work. The relevant chapter is clearly an abridged version of what his teacher had written on the subject.

CHAPTER 3

The Renaissance

In the middle of the fifteenth century a cultural change took place in Europe which was so revolutionary that it may well be said that a new era had dawned. The contempt of worldliness shown by mediaeval man, who saw the fulfilment of his existence in the hereafter, gave way to the realization that life on earth is also very worthwhile.

This new attitude enhanced interest in man and the world in which he lives. Prompted by curiosity, many set sail to see what was beyond the horizon, others pointed the newly invented telescope at the night sky, yet others opened the human body to inspect its inner construction.

The rise of anatomy, in which of course Andreas Vesalius (1514–64) of Brussels played a paramount part, in its turn stimulated the development of surgery. Surgery owed its revival, however, just as much to the wars which devastated the Old World in the sixteenth and seventeenth centuries: quite a few of the Renaissance surgeons had acquired their experience and their manual skill on the battle-fields. As to the theoretical conceptions of disease, changes were less spectacular. The views of Galen and other authors from antiquity remained unquestioned; humoralism still dominated the medical mind.

One of the most prominent members of these generations of surgeons who helped to shape a new surgery was without doubt Ambroise Paré (1510–90), surgeon to four successive French kings. Amongst other things, he may be given credit for the reintroduction of vascular ligature, which had fallen into disuse in the Middle Ages. His books on anatomy and surgery were read all over Europe. In his *Oeuvres complètes* of 1575 an important chapter occurs on 'Tumeurs contre nature'.[44] True to the Galenic tradition, he understood by 'tumeurs' inflammations, skin diseases, oedema and other unnatural swellings apart from scirrhus and carcinoma. Paré's views on the aetiology of malignant tumours are representative for Renaissance oncology. These views, however, were better explained by Paré's contemporary Falloppio, whose work is discussed later in this chapter. Paré's clinical description of malignant breast disease, in which he made mention of inflammations and swellings of the glands in the axilla, was derived from Aetius, that is to say from Archigenes and Leonides. His modes of treatment, conservative as well as surgical, are not much different from those of Galen. To promote the patient's peace of mind, he advises her against gossiping with other women. There are a few additions, however. From the *Practica in arte chirurgica copiosa* written by the papal court physician Giovanni da Vigo (1460?–1517?), Paré took a mercury ointment for the external treatment of scirrhus. In cases of ulcerated cancer he recommended, among many other things, the application of a puppy, a kitten or any other young animal, cut in two lengthwise. After the animal's body had cooled, it should be replaced by a fresh one.[45] We often have occasion to note, especially in the treatment of cancer, that old therapeutic methods, having been abolished by official medicine, linger on in so-called folk-medicine or in quackery. As late as 1924, an Amsterdam quack was convicted of having split open a live puppy to apply it to breast cancer.[46]

Paré's works derive their charm in particular from the numerous case-histories that enliven the text. Thus he recalled the case of Madame de Montigny, a lady-in-waiting to the queen-mother, who consulted him on a tender lump, as big as a walnut, in her left breast. Paré's diagnosis was cancer, but he thought it advisable not to inform the patient. With the approval of the lady's medical consultant, he restricted his therapy to purging and to the local application of a lead sheet smeared over with mercury ointment. While it was true that in the next two months there was no worsening, there was no improvement either. However, the patient became impatient and placed herself under the treatment of a physician who had promised her a certain cure. He applied irritating heating and absorbing medicines with the disastrous result that the tumour rapidly increased in size and did not take long to burst open like a ripe pomegranate. Repeated haemorrhages ultimately led to the death of the patient. 'And in such a way, the physician had fulfilled his promise to cure her. He did in fact not only cure her of her present disease, but of all the ailments of this world', concluded Paré.[47]

It may strike the reader that in this case-history the patient was presented under her full name. This occurred often in medical literature of that time. Indeed, professional secrecy, although an essential item of the ancient and venerable Hippocratic oath, was not generally observed in medical publications until the middle of the nineteenth century.

Case-histories, hardly encountered in the medical literature of the Middle Ages, became rapidly popular in the Renaissance and collected clinical observations occupied an important place in the scientific output of the period. A specimen of this type of literature is Fabricius' *Observationum et curationum chirurgicarum centuriae*. The author, Wilhelm Fabry (1560–1634) of Hilden, was the most outstanding German surgeon of his time. He believed that cancer begins with a drop of milk curdling within the breast. One of Fabry's surgical feats was the removal of bulky swellings in the armpit in a case of breast cancer. To that purpose he made an incision over the swellings, took one node out with his finger nails and had a second tumour seized with a small forceps and drawn out from the depth by an assistant. He then cut it loose between two stitch ligatures, applied with a curved needle. The ends of the central ligature were carried out at the wound, as was common practice in pre-antiseptic times, to await their spontaneous expulsion. Thereupon he excised the diseased breast in the usual manner with a separate incision.[48]

The exact nature of the usual manner is clearly shown in the familiar picture in the book by Scultetus (Johann Schultes, 1595–1645), a German surgeon in Ulm[49] (Fig. 9). The Amazonian operation as such was not conceived by Scultetus himself, it had

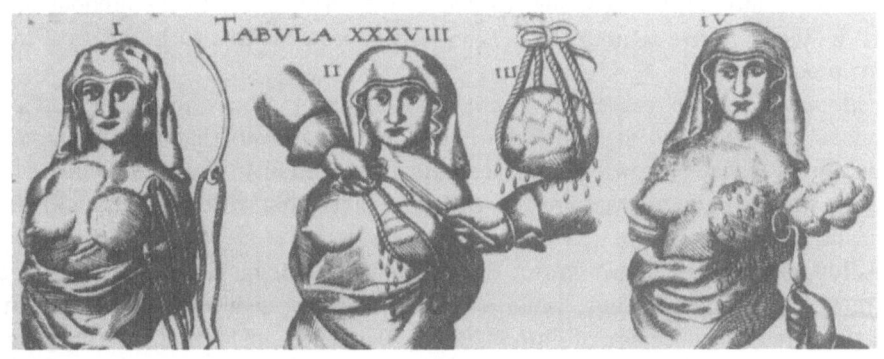

Fig. 9.   Mastectomy in the 16th and 17th centuries.

already been described by the widely renowned Spanish surgeon Francisco Arceo
(1493?–15?) in 1574.[50]

An extensive discussion on scirrhus and cancer, representative for the sixteenth
century, appeared in the surgical works of Gabriele Falloppio (1523–62).[51] Falloppio
is still remembered as an anatomist – tubae Falloppii – but he was also a first-rate
surgeon. During the last years of his short life he occupied the combined chairs of
anatomy, surgery and botany at the renowned university of Padua. His surgical tracts
appeared only after his death. Edited by former students, they clearly bear the
character of lectures. In his humoralistic views on the genesis of malignant growths,
Falloppio was a confirmed Galenist. He did accept the existence of two kinds of black
bile, however, a natural and a non-natural species. Non-natural bile did not originate in
the liver as did the natural variety, but was a 'combustion product' of other humours
as was already explained by Henri de Mondeville some three centuries earlier.[52] In
spite of the considerable lapse of time that separated them, Falloppio counted Henri
de Mondeville among the 'iuniores', together with Guglielmo, Bruno, Teodorico, Guy
and the like. These mediaeval surgeons probably owed their age-old juniorship to
the fact that after them no important new theories were proposed in the field of
oncology.

The material cause of scirrhus and cancer was always a fluxion of a sluggish, thick
humour. According to the composition of the humour in question, which could be
either of the two atrabiliary humours whether or not admixed with phlegm, yellow
bile or blood, there were different grades of malignancy. The addition of cold phlegm
resulted in scirrhous tumours of a relatively benign character, whereas the presence of
blood should be looked upon as highly ominous since blood was endowed with the
elementary quality of 'heat'. Heat predisposed to inflammation, a blend of melancholic
humour, especially of the burnt kind, and blood therefore meant the most dangerous
combination thinkable since it would produce inflammatory cancer. Ulceration
pointed to putrefaction of the melancholic compound.[53]

The above makes it clear why Renaissance surgeons attached so much importance
to dietary measures by way of treatment. Diet should be devoid of 'hot' elements,

should preferably even be cooling, to add as little as possible to the noxious factor 'heat' in the causative tumour. Even blood-letting now appears to be a logical therapeutic procedure.

Falloppio's remote causes were not very different from those that had been advanced ever since the days of Galen. He admits, however, that the true mode of origin is not always known and he accepts the possibility of an iatrogenic cause, namely, when the doctor has treated an innocent tumour with the wrong kinds of medicine.[52]

Falloppio's clinical description of the affected breast is more detailed than Paré's. Scirrhus is basically indolent; when a tumour becomes painful it means that it is changing into cancer because of putrefaction of the 'succus melancholicus'. Irregularity is a sure sign of malignancy, whereas swollen veins are not as typical as is generally believed. The tumour may be adherent to the pectoral muscles, in which case it is inoperable.[54]

The Padua professor was highly conservative in his treatment of breast cancer. Quiet cancers should be left in peace.[54] Mastectomy is only indicated in some cases of ulceration, the operation should be performed according to Leonides, quoted by Aetius. Amongst the many medicines for local applications, he particularly recommends round marine or fresh-water crabs, burnt to ashes or cooked in milk; there is nothing better for ulcerated cancers. If, however, the pain cannot be allayed 'tunc rogandus est Deus, ut vita aegrum privet' (then the Lord should be asked to take the patient's life).[53]

Although it was realized at the time that mammary cancer may be accompanied by swellings in the axilla, not much thought was, as yet, being given to the phenomenon of metastasis.

The new morphological approach to the human body, as evidenced by the steadily increasing interest in anatomy ever since the sixteenth century, also gave rise to speculations on the nature of matter. It was surely not the first time in history that such fundamental questions had been pondered. In the fifth or sixth century B.C. the Greek natural philosopher Demokritus of Abdera had taught that all material things in existence are composed of countless infinitesimal and indivisible solid particles, of varying shape, in perpetual motion. From this primitive atomism, a tendency of thought had developed that strongly competed with humoral pathology in ancient medicine. This school's doctrines were that the solid parts of the body consist of cohesive particles. Within the mass, a network of tiny interstices would have been left. Through these 'pores', the body fluids would percolate, these fluids themselves being composed of minute solid particles. Any incongruity between the diameter of the 'pores' and the size of the fluid particles would either slow down or accelerate the flow, and in either case disease would ensue.[55]

It was Galen who, in the competitive struggle between humoral and solidistic pathology, gained the mastery in late antiquity. After having been buried in oblivion for many centuries, ancient materialism was revived in the beginning of the seventeenth century by Prosper Alpinus (1553—1617). It is perhaps no mere coincidence that Alpinus was professor of medicine at Padua in Italy, where Galileo Galilei, one of the founders of modern mechanics, was his contemporary and anatomy as an academic discipline was strongly represented ever since the beginning of the sixteenth century.

The renewed acquaintanceship with the ideal world of the ancient solidistic pathologists did not imply that humoralism was immediately abandoned in favour of solidism. Still, some basic thoughts were borrowed from the rival doctrine, among others, the useful notion that the blocking of pores — now conceived as obstruction of blood vessels and other anatomical duct systems — would give rise to all sorts of diseases. We will return to this later. The discovery of blood circulation — mainly a hydrodynamic process — by William Harvey in 1628 greatly contributed to the new tendency to explain physiological processes in health and disease by the laws of mechanics.

Not all physicians, however, were happy with the modern iatromechanical trend in medicine. They were not prepared to look upon the body as a machine as Descartes had suggested and to regard its functions as mechanical processes. Influenced by another branch of science then arising, there were many who preferred to explain physiological phenomena by chemical categories.

A leading member of this 'iatrochemical school' was the Leyden professor François de le Boë Sylvius (1614–72), a Frenchman by birth (Fig. 10). In his pathophysiological considerations Sylvius attached great importance to lymph. His preoccupation was quite modern: the lymphatic system had only just been discovered and anatomists vied with one another in describing its details. It was Thomas Bartholin of Copenhagen (1616–80), a member of a family of distinguished anatomists, who in 1653 had introduced the designation 'vasa lymphatica' for the newly discovered systems of vessels.[56] The Latin word 'lympha' (clear spring water) was suggested to him on account of the clear, watery contents of these vessels. Bartholin believed that lymph was derived from blood through a process of straining or filtration. The word 'lymphaticus' was not entirely new, though. It occurs already in classical literature, signifying insane, beside oneself. It was likewise derived from lympha, but then from 'lympha'/'nymph'. Something of the ominous emotional value of being seized by nasty nymphs, seems to have lingered in the seventeenth-century use of the word lymph.

Lymph was, as Sylvius had established by tasting, a 'succus subacidus', a subacid juice. Should, however, the slightly acid nature turn into acrid acid, the ensuing 'acrimony', sharp and biting in nature, would give rise to morbid conditions.[57] The pathological principle of acrimony, although a chemical concept, was also accepted by the 'iatromechanics'. The latter, of course, tried to define acrimony on mechanical tenets. Fluid particles would carry hooks or would look like needles which, in certain circumstances, could damage the walls of the conducting vessels, producing the pain that iatrochemists chose to explain in terms of 'acid quality'. The microscopical observation of Antoni van Leeuwenhoek (1632–1723), who had seen minute pointed particles in drying vinegar, which appeared to explain the sharp and acid taste of it, seemed to affirm the views of the iatromechanics. The more so, since the same microscopist had observed similar formations in urine which proved that sharp particles do indeed occur in the living body.[58] Such were, in outline, the main new pathogenetic concepts which appeared in medical literature during the approximately 200 years

Fig. 10. Professor François de le Boë Sylvius.

that constituted the transition period between the gradual abandonment of Galenic humoral pathology, starting in the seventeenth century, and the acceptance of cellular pathology some 125 years ago. Widely divergent as the lines of thought seem to be, the categories lymph, acid, acrimony, corrosion, stasis and coagulation may be met in most of them.

Iatrochemists and iatrophysicists agreed that cancer had its origin in lymph, rather than in any natural or non-natural black bile, but held divergent views on how exactly malignant growths developed from lymph. Sylvius, the iatrochemist, taught that cancer would result when 'tempered' acid turned into 'acrid' acid: 'ab acido enim acri cancrum generari'.[59] Friedrich Hoffmann (1660–1742), professor of medicine in Halle and one of the most authoritative medical authors towards the end of the century, may be cited as a partisan of the iatromechanical school of thought. He imputed cancer to coagulation of lymph, brought about by obstruction of the lymph flow. An uncomplicated stagnation would cause 'scirrhus', but if a 'corrosive acid substance' came into play, the outcome would be 'carcinoma'.[60] The corrosive element explained why, in contrast to scirrhus, carcinoma is so often so extremely painful.

22

The introduction of contemporary lymphatic theories did not mean, however, that the traditional role of black bile was entirely discarded: ancient and modern theories coexisted all through the seventeenth and eighteenth centuries, sometimes even becoming entwined. Pierre Dionis (1643–1718) cited three different authors defending different views. Dionis was an outstanding Paris surgeon, whose anatomical and surgical lectures and demonstrations in the Jardin des Plantes attracted numerous attendants from all over Europe. His *Course d'opérations de chirurgie* (1707) was translated into several languages.[61] To two of them, Jean-Baptiste Alliot (?–1729) and Claude-Deshais Gendron (1663–1750) he apparently assigned some authority on the grounds that the father of the one and the uncle of the other had been involved – be it in vain – in the treatment of the mammary cancer of Anne of Austria, mother of the reigning King Louis XIV. This royal sick-bed will be referred to below.

Jean-Baptiste Alliot, physician to the Bastille prison in Paris, held that scirrhus developed from black bile, but could contain some acid as well. Should this acid get the upper hand of the salt in the blood, scirrhus would turn into carcinoma. The pain by which carcinoma distinguished itself from scirrhus was brought about by the sharp pines and barbs of the acid particles.[62]

A different explanation was given by Claude-Deshais Gendron, personal physician to royalty and the central figure of a cultural circle in the French capital. He described malignant growth as 'nerve-like and gland-like parts' which had turned, together with lymph vessels, into an even, cold, homogenous mass in which the original elements are no longer recognizable. It spreads along 'filamens durs', which it sends into the adjoining parts. These solid protrusions are the real 'cancer roots', not the dilated veins of the ancients. Gendron's nosological concept was clearly solidistic; in this respect it stands somewhat alone until the middle of the eighteenth century.[63]

The third author quoted by Dionis was Adrian Helvetius (1661–1741).[64] This Dutch physician from The Hague, whose real family name was Schweitzer, enjoyed a great reputation in the French capital since he had cured the Dauphin of dysentery by means of ipecacuanha root, recently introduced from Brazil. He boasted that his father had extirpated more than two thousand breast cancers in The Hague. The Paris surgeon Jean Devaux (1649–1729), who mentioned this extravagant claim in a supplement to his *Index funereus chirurgicorum*, dryly remarked that it was not 'un article de foy' (an article of faith).[65] Helvetius held the view that cancer begins with a drop of fluid coagulating within a gland. A 'ferment' would be influential in the further expansion of the process. The cause of the primordial coagulation he held to be in most cases some form of external trauma: a blow, a fall and the like. In an early stage, the lesion could be made to dissolve by means of caustic chemicals; once the tumour had set hard it was better not to 'irritate' it with such remedies since the effect might be quite the opposite. He gave, however, no definition of the early stage. Helvetius was in favour of operative therapy: by excision when the lesion was still small, by amputation when the growth was extensive and in a state of ulceration.

Dionis showed himself a follower of both Hoffman and Sylvius in attributing the origin of cancer to the stagnation of lymph in the breast, followed by inspissation and souring. The stasis could be brought about either by external trauma, or by noxious 'earthlike' constituents of blood loaded with acid material. Dionis accepted the ancient view of some sort of relation existing between the uterus and the breast, since most patients are between forty and sixty years old when they contract the disease. When struck at a younger age, they usually are 'pas bien réglées'. Among his patients were many nuns. Dionis also acknowledged the influence of the mind. Since sorrow or anger could bring about coagulation of humours, the sufferers should be encouraged to adopt a cheerful attitude. Cheerfulness and good humour further 'soft fermentation' of the blood and an even distribution of vital spirits.[66] Before proceeding to a mastectomy, Dionis used to mark the lines of incision with ink.

In the seventeenth century medical literature, frequent mention is made of enlarged and hardened glands in the ipsilateral axilla. The cause of these enlargements was thought to be the same as the one underlying the lump in the breast. Contemporary autopsy reports with a clear description of visceral dissemination are lacking, to my knowledge. No definite explanation of the cause of death in cases of cancer was given either: there was some vague notion of a poison secreted by the afflicted parts. Belief in the existence of a particular cancer poison grew stronger, however, as the century progressed.

A question that would remain unsettled for quite some time to come concerned the possible contagiousness of cancer, of the ulcerating type in particular. Amongst those who considered the disease to be infectious was the Amsterdam physician and anatomist Nicholas Tulp (1593–1674), who was immortalized by Rembrandt in his famous 'Anatomical Lesson'. In support of his view, Tulp cited the case of his patient Adriana Lamberta, an elderly lady suffering from open breast cancer, who was thought to have conveyed the disease to her housemaid.[67] Since scientific communications were mostly written in Latin at the time and medical books were slow to become obsolete, the misfortune of the two Amsterdam women served for a long time as a positive proof all over Europe. This illustrates how, even in the seventeenth and eighteenth centuries, a single observation could be accepted as conclusive evidence. The history of scientific medicine is to no small extent a history of the handling of evidence.

The belief in the contagiousness of cancer persisted until well into the nineteenth century in medical and legislative minds, and even today traces of the old anxiety seem to linger amongst patients and their relatives. In the seventeenth and eighteenth centuries, cancer patients were not, in some places, admitted to public hospitals.[68] It is possible, however, that an etching by Rembrandt represents a woman admitted to an Amsterdam hospital with a cancer of her right breast[69] (Fig. 11).

As before, therapy was either conservative, prescribing diet, purges, blood letting and medicines, or surgical. Those physicians and surgeons who attached importance to 'acidity' were, of course, inclined to prescribe alkaline drugs. Thus Alliot lauded an alkaline arsenic, to be applied on cancer sores. As often happens in the history of medicine, an old remedy — arsenic, in this case — was made to fit a new theory. Gendron, on the other hand, had no use for 'acid-breaking' remedies since in his solidistic view it was the protusions of the growth, rather than 'acidity', that caused incurability. Such a view of course encouraged surgery.

Non-operative treatment seems to have been the rule in early stages since patients and surgeons alike flinched from the ordeal of intervention. This was apparently the

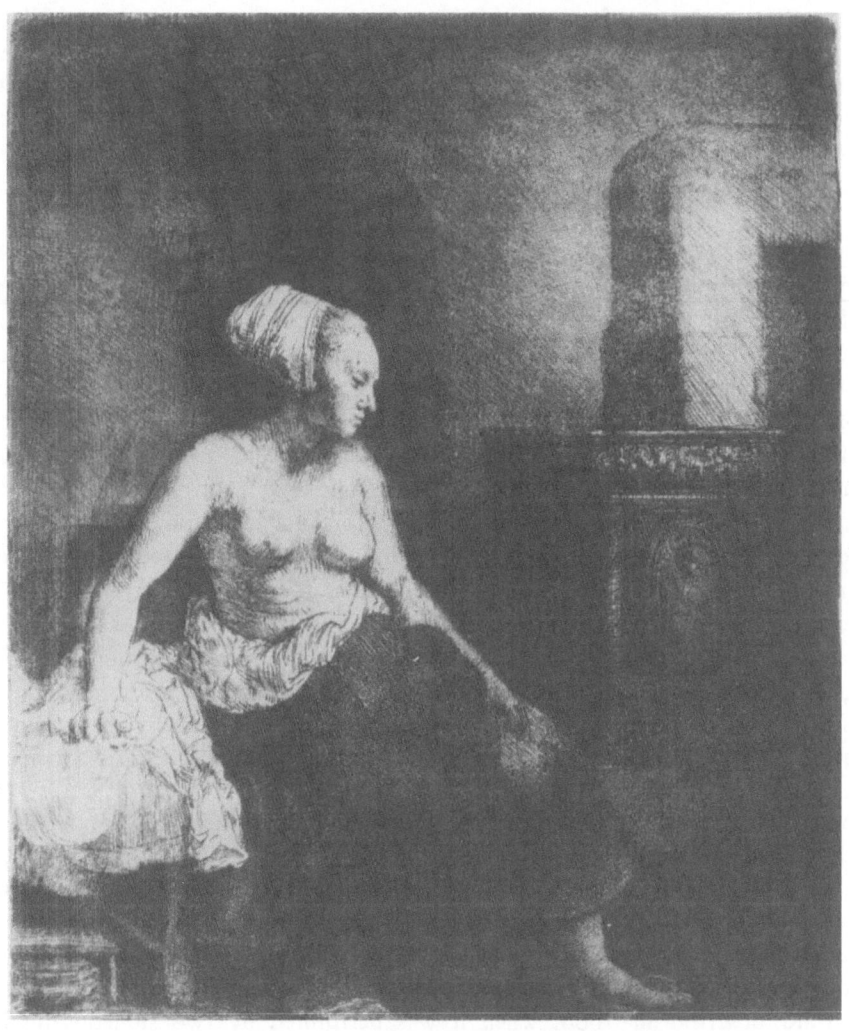

Fig. 11. Rembrandt: Woman sitting half-dressed beside a stove.

case when in the spring of 1664 Anne of Austria, mother of King Louis XIV of France, sent for her personal physician to examine a small, solid nodule in her left breast. That worthy dignitary, Pierre Seguin (1566–1623), immediately recognized its true character, but wisely abstained from any therapy, perhaps bearing Hippocrates' sound advice in mind. The Queen-mother now treated her diseased breast, on the advice of her maids, with compresses saturated in the juice of hemlock. This was continued until the end of the year, but the lump steadily increased in size, whereas the patient grew weaker and weaker, while her face took on a yellowish tinge.

The personal physician of the King, Antoine Vallot (1594–1671), was next consulted. He substituted ointments for the compresses, but before long the breast burst open and a huge ulcer appeared. It was clear that regular medicine had nothing more to offer and, as so often happens in such desperate cases, a quack was called in. This happened to be an uncle of Claude-Deshais Gendron, whom we discussed previously. The elder Gendron was a Roman-Catholic priest, who had a number of miraculous cures to his credit. His secret remedy – containing belladonna, as was later disclosed by his physician-nephew – was, however, of no avail. In the meanwhile, the Queen's right arm swelled and an abscess formed in the axilla, necessitating an incision. Although some pus was let out, sizable protuberances remained.

Then another performer of cancer cures was sent for, a doctor this time, practising in the small provincial town of Bar-le-Duc. This was Pierre Alliot (?–1680), father of Jean-Baptiste Alliot, whose eclectic views on cancer we have already considered. Alliot senior, in his turn, applied a remedy of secret composition. This appeared to be a caustic, containing arsenic as turned out afterwards. The necrotic parts were daily cut off in the presence of the royal family, the physicians and surgeons of the court and other members of the royal household. This treatment had to be discontinued because of intolerable pain. Other practitioners followed, from places as far apart as Milan in Italy and Oirschot in The Netherlands. Before embarking on surgical treatment of breast cancer the Oirschot surgeon, Arnoldus Fey (?–1679), used to issue a legal document declaring that he could not be held liable for any untoward results or for the failure of his efforts.[70] It is not known what treatment Fey suggested.

It was clear that the royal patient was beyond help, however. She suffered atrocious pains, the ulcer gave off a foul and penetrating smell and both her arms, her shoulders and her neck were affected with erysipelas. After a prolonged agony she expired on January 20th 1666, some twenty months after the appearance of the first symptoms of the disease.[71]

Operative treatment found a staunch advocate in the physician Tulp: 'Unicum remedium est, tempestiva sectio' (the sole remedy is a timely operation), he emphasised. Some surgeons cut off the breast in one swift sweeping movement with a big razor. Others used their fingers to detach the mammary gland bluntly from the thoracic wall, entering via a preliminary incision, until in the end only a rim of skin had to be cut. It was apparently a variety of this type of operation which the Reverend John Ward observed in 1666, when it was performed by two surgeons on Mrs. Townsend, one of his parishioners in Stratford-on-Avon:[72]

First they cutt the skin cross and laid itt back, then they workt their hands in ytt, one above and the other below, and so till their hands mett, and so brought itt out. They had their needles and waxt thread ready, but never ust them; and allso their cauterizing irons, but they used them not: she lost not above six ounces of blood in all. Dr. Needham coming too late, staid next day to see it opened. Hee said itt was a melliceris (a cystic tumour filled with a honey-like substance), and not a perfect cancer; but itt would have been one quickly. There came out a gush of a great quantitie of waterish substance, as much as would fill a flaggon; when they had done, they cutt off, one one bitt, another another, and putt in a glass of wine and some lint, and so let itt alone till the next day; then they opend itt again, and injected myrrhe, aloes, and such things as resisted putrefaction, and so bound itt upp againe. Every time they dresst itt, they cutt off something of the cancer

26

that was left behind; the chyrurgions were for applying a caustick, but Dr. Needham said no, not till the last, since shee could endure the knife. They prepard her bodie somewhat, and let her blood the day before. One of the chyrurgeons told her afterwards, that shee had endured soe much, that hee would have lost his life ere hee would have sufferd the like; and the Dr. said hee had read that women would endure more than men, but did not beleeve itt till now. The way how and where itt should bee cutt was markt with ink by one Dr. Edwards, who lives at Bridgnorth, Mrs Townsend likt him very well; hee said iff they could prevent a gangrene there was little fear, iff shee fell not into a feavour.

1666. Mrs. Townsend, of Alverston, being dead of a cancer, Mr. Eedes and I opened her breast in the outward part, and fount itt very cancrous; itt had been broken, and a mellicerous part was yet remaining when wee saw itt, which being launct, yielded two porringers full of a very yellow substance, which came out plentifully out of the cavities of the breast. The flesh that was growne againe, after part was taken out, was of a hard gristly substance, which seemed very strange. The ribbs were not putrefied as wee could discerne, not anything within the breast of a cancrous nature, for wee runne the knife withinside the breast through the intercostal muscles. Dr. Needham hath affirmed that a cancer is as much within as without the breast, and hee hath seen a string, as I was told, going from the breast to the uterus. I suppose itt was the mammillarie veins full of knotts which were cancrous, and hung much like ropes of onions. The cancer was a strange one, as was evident; wee wanted spunges and other things convenient, or else wee had opened the cavitie of the breast.

The etching by the Dutch painter and illustrator Romeyn de Hooghe (1695–1708) depicts how a mastectomy would have been performed round about 1667 (Fig. 12). This was, at least, the year in which the book appeared from which this illustration was taken. This work is not a medical treatise, however, but a collection of emblems: pictures with a succint caption relating to the moral lesson symbolized in the illustration. It is entitled *Voorhof der Ziele* (Forecourt of the Soul). The sixty fine etchings are all executed by the same artist. The accompanying lines, composed by the Rotterdam bookseller François van Hoogstraten, are of an edifying nature. As appears from the dedication and eulogies printed in front, the righteous bookshop-owner felt that he should convert his fellowmen to virtue and piety. The text under the depiction of a mastectomy was inspired by the second epistle to Timothy (2, verses 16 and 17), in which Paul expresses his disapproval of godless people whose 'word will eat as does the canker'. This epistle is the only place in the Bible in which there is an explicit reference to cancer. The harm done by the books of certain objectionable authors is compared by van Hoogstraten to the proliferation of a malignant growth in the physical body. Just as a cancer can only be cured by timely application of a 'sharp knife', so errant souls must be restored to the straight and narrow path by painful correction. This kind of figurative language had already been used by the Greek Father of the Church Johannes Chrysostomos, patriarch of Constantinople (345–407 A.D.).

The vivid representation by Romeyn de Hooghe is undoubtedly taken from reality. The drama is enacted in the presence of the husband and two weeping daughters

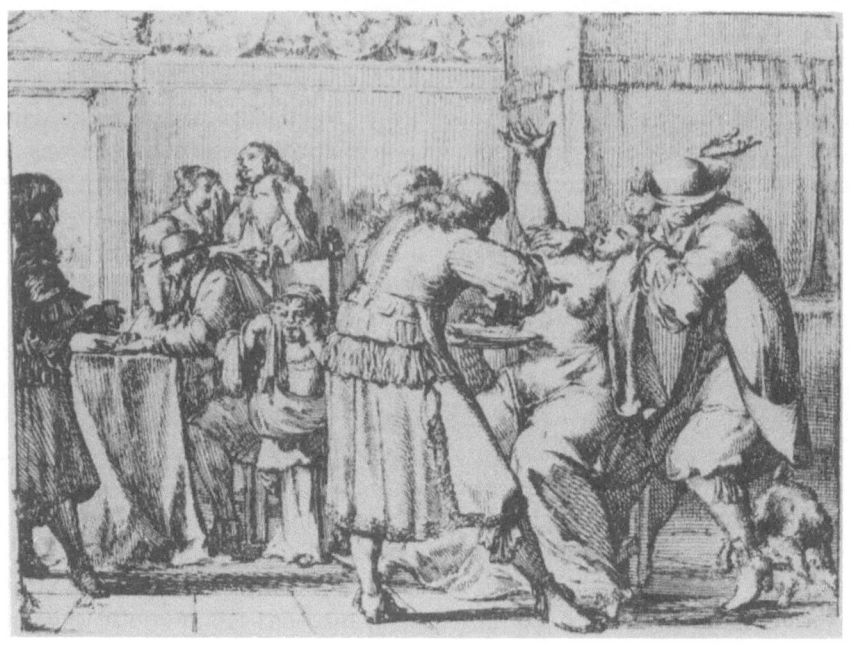

Fig. 12.   Romeyn de Hooghe: mastectomy.

in the patient's own bedroom: until late in the nineteenth century hospitals were intended only for paupers. The patient is sitting on a chair opposite the surgeon who is engaged in removing the diseased organ. She is held down by an assistant, while a second helper catches the blood, which — almost invisible to the spectator — spurts forth from the wound. The arm at the stricken side is abducted and elevated to tighten the pectoral muscle, exactly as is recommended in the textbooks of the period. At a table sits the doctor of medicine without whose presence no surgeon was allowed to perform a major operation. Dignified and unmoved he wields his pen, presumably to prescribe a diet and appropriate medicines. The person standing in front of him is probably the apothecary, holding a mug which might have contained a cordial.[73]

Detailed descriptions of excision of the breast by eyewitnesses such as Reverend Ward are very rare indeed. If any such operations are ever mentioned at all in non-medical sources, they are often referred to in passing, as, for instance, by Samuel Pepys when he casually entered the following in his diary on May 5th, 1665: 'My wife tells me that she hears that my poor aunt James hath had her breast cut off here in town, her breast having long been out of order'.

We may well ask whether operative treatment was adopted at the time on a large scale at all. The average duration of life was only 35 years, so that comparatively few women will have reached the age at which breast cancer occurs most frequently. Gripping scenes, such as those described by Ward and depicted by de Hooghe, will not particularly have encouraged women to call in medical aid as soon as they felt a lump.

Yet the Leyden Professor Johannes van Horne (1621–70) stated that breast amputation was a common intervention in his day. He gave no specific information, however.[74] Figures hardly had a place in medical thinking before late in the eighteenth century.

His younger contemporary in The Hague, the M.D.-surgeon Govert Bidloo (1649–1713), famous for his magnificent anatomical atlas with illustrations by Gerard de Lairesse, casually remarked that in 1679 he had performed that operation twenty times within a single year. He did not give any particulars as to the results.[75] Much later, his former pupil Hendrik Ulhoorn (1692?–1749), a well-known surgeon in Amsterdam, whom we will discuss in the next chapter, stated that in his youth he had attended many of Bidloo's operations, 'but since the great man did not pay particular attention to the difficulties cited just now, we witnessed but few happy outcomes of his work'.[76] Ulhoorn is here referring to the rules regarding operability and inoperability that were being formulated towards the end of the seventeenth century, when it became clear that the presence of axillary nodes and adherence to the ribs should preclude amputation.

The huge wound was treated with salves and other materials which could prevent bandages from sticking to its surface. Secondary haemorrhage was the most dreaded, directly postoperative complication. Such an event could only be treated by a compression bandage, if need be with an inverted soup plate bound over it to prevent the seepage of blood. Morgagni mentioned the danger of 'febriles accessiones', accompanying inflammation, which could cause the death of the patient.[77] In the absence of serious complications, the amputation wound could heal by granulation within a few months.

The patient was usually considered cured as soon as her wound had healed. Very few surgeons reported on their late results. Richard Wiseman (1622–76), surgeon to King Charges II and the author of a very popular textbook, remarked that only two patients out of a series of twelve breast cancer cases were definitely cured by mastectomy. One of them was only 20 years old. Two others died after the operation, the eight others expired under conservative treatment.[78] Bidloo reported that one of his patients had lived for five years, despite having an ulcerating wound with excrescences that had to be cut away regularly.[75]

The first surgeon to aim at healing by direct union was 'a certain empiric' in Berlin in 1698. His patient was a French refugee lady, belonging to the important Huguenot colony in the Prussian capital. After having transfixed the lump to secure a grip, he performed a large excision. The elliptiform wound was closed with five stitches. Soon afterwards it became inflamed and started to produce a foul matter. Glandules appeared in the armpit and the arm became swollen to the wrist. The woman suffered excruciating pain and expired after some ten weeks. A limited post-mortem showed that a cancerous process had formed in the wound, which had penetrated the chest wall and extended also across the sternum to the other breast.[79] Gustav Casimir Gahrliep van der Müllen (1630–1717), an outstanding Berlin physician, who reported on this case in the *Ephemerides naturae curiosorum*, attributed the fateful outcome to closure of the wound before a correct amount of blood, loaded as it was with 'souring disease' (acorescatens aegritudo), had escaped. This case was repeatedly referred to in later discussions on the question of whether, after excision, the wound should be closed or left open.

The *Ephemerides*, or *Miscellanea curiosa medico-physica academiae naturae curiosorum sive ephemeridum medico-physicarum germanicarum curiosarum*, as the official title goes, was a mainly medical and biological periodical first issued in 1670 under the auspices of one of the earliest scientific societies, the 'Academia Naturae Curiosorum'. Both academy and periodical still exist. Scientific journals started to play a part — for some time, only a modest one — in medical communication late in the seventeenth century.

CHAPTER 4

Pathophysiological concepts
in the Age of Enlightenment

In many ways the eighteenth century was also an Age of Enlightenment for surgery. Towards the end of the century, the steady improvements being made in clinical diagnosis as well as in operative techniques based on accurate anatomical knowledge, together with the development of sophisticated tools, had raised the practice of surgery to the highest conceivable level which could be reached without asepsis and anaesthesia. The traditional social differences between surgeons and physicians dwindled as more and more surgeons took a medical degree and the teaching of surgery gradually assumed a more scientific and clinical character. The latter applied in particular to France and the United Kingdom.

In Paris and London large hospitals began to allow practical and theoretical training on a hitherto unprecedented scale. Paris in particular had much to offer to surgical students: there were public and private lectures in anatomy and operative surgery in the anatomical theatres, in the Jardin des Plantes du Roy and elsewhere, and clinical demonstrations of numerous surgical cases in the teaching hospitals. Jean-Louis Petit (1674–1750), Henri-François le Dran (1685–1770), Prudent Hevin (1715–89), François Quesnay (1694–1774) and, somewhat later, Antoine Louis (1723–1792), were the leading Paris surgeons of their day. Henri-François de Dran was one of the sixteen children of Henri le Dran (1656–1720), a Paris surgeon who had revived the operation of mastectomy in France, after it had long been neglected[65] (Fig. 13). In Rouen, Claude-Nicholas le Cat (1700–1768) enjoyed an international reputation. In 1731, the Académie de Chirurgie was founded. The *Mémoires*, published by that distinguished society, was the first periodical entirely devoted to surgery: for thirty years it embodied the vanguard of surgical knowledge in Europe. Scientific surgery was also promoted by prizes, offered by learned bodies like universities and academies all over Europe. Although in France and elsewhere, in the second half of the eighteenth century in particular, laboratory experiments were sometimes resorted to in the study of cancer, pathophysiological concepts remained highly speculative.

In London, where, as everywhere else, surgeons and barbers had been organized in Barber-Surgeon's Guilds, the surgeons separated from the barbers in 1745. A new era in surgery was ushered into British surgery by William Cheselden (1688–1752), surgeon to the St. Thomas' and St. George's Hospitals. He was the first to establish private courses in anatomy and surgery. Many distinguished surgeon-anatomists, like the Hunter brothers, followed suit. Such courses attracted students from all over the

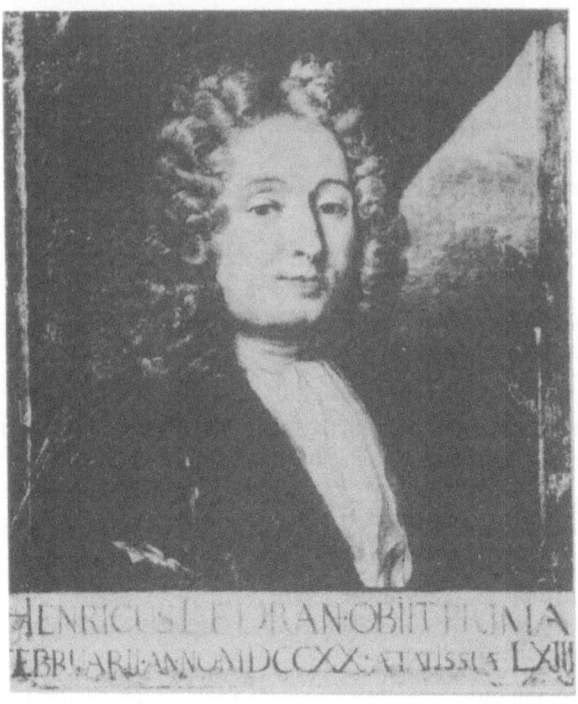

Fig. 13. Henri-François le Dran.

country and even from the continent. A great surgeon active at the time in London was the Scot John Hunter (1728–93) (Fig. 14). John Hunter is particularly remembered as the founder of experimental surgery and surgical pathology.

In Edinburgh the separation of the surgeons from the barbers was for practical purposes complete from 1718. In that city the scene was, in contrast to London, dominated by university teachers, more in particular by successive members of the Monro family.

A more modest centre of surgery existed in Amsterdam, where in the eighteenth century anatomists and surgeons like Frederik Ruysch (1638–1731), Hendrik Ulhoorn and Petrus Camper (1722–89) attracted students also from other countries, especially Germany.

On the whole, German surgery lagged behind somewhat in the eighteenth century. The textbooks of Lorenz Heister (1683–1758), professor in Altdorf and Helmstedt, successively, and of August Gottlieb Richter (1742–1812) in Göttingen, did much to remedy that situation. In Vienna, Gerard van Swieten (1700–72) should be recalled in particular, not only because he was the founder of the famous medical school in the Austrian capital, but also because he translated and commented upon the *Aphorisms* of his preceptor professor Herman Boerhaave (1668–1738) in Leyden, who had enjoyed a world-wide reputation as a clinical teacher.

The eighteenth century produced a number of fundamental dissertations on the aetiology of cancer, together with many detailed case histories; yet essential

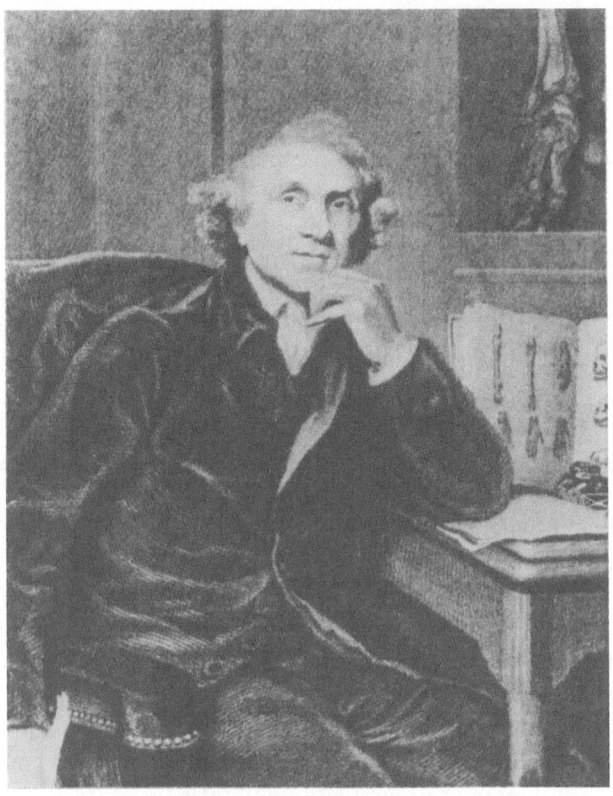

Fig. 14. John Hunter.

developments in pathophysiological concepts were slow to occur. In many textbooks of the period – and even of the early nineteenth century – all sorts of tumefacient morbid conditions, varying from skin diseases to scrofula, cancer, varicose veins and aneurysms, can be found under the heading of 'Preternatural Tumours'. The Galenic distinction between scirrhus and carcinoma remained in force, some authorities considering scirrhus to be a separate, basically benign growth which, under adverse conditions, might undergo malignant degeneration, whilst other simply regarded it as a stage of cancer. The rapid progression of the disease once it had eroded the skin was attributed by Le Cat,[80] Hevin[81] and others to the putrefying properties of air which now had full access to the pathological process. It appears that, long before Pasteur and Lister, surgeons connected wound inflammation with free access of air.[82] Scirrhus was still thought by the vast majority of medical people to have its immediate origin in stagnation and coagulation of body fluids in the mammary gland. Coagulation could have a local cause, but it could also be brought about by an internal derangement of the body juices. Almost all authors accepted both origins, either occurring separately or acting conjointly. In the latter case, a local cause would only be a precipitating factor in a predisposed patient.

Local causes were mainly of a mechanical nature: a bruise as a result of a fall or a blow, pressure caused by garments like the tight bodice introduced by Madame de Pompadour, the application of medicines or compresses. Boerhaave's opinion: 'Nam contusio quae in cute nullius momenti esset, eadem in glandula conglomerata scirrhum pessimum producit' (For a contusion that would be of no importance to the skin, produces the worst scirrhus in a compound gland),[83] was cited with approval by Morgagni, who could offer an example from his personal experience.[77] Milk, curdled within the breast, could also act as a physical agent by compressing vessels. The well-known Paris surgeon and obstetrician Jean Astruc (1684–1766) advanced yet another mechanical cause when he put the blame on 'la facilité qu'on a de se laisser prendre et manier les tetons, ce qui les expose à des compressions' (The complaisance with which nowadays one allows one's teats to be taken and handled, exposing them to compression...).[84] Astruc unwittingly confirmed an observation expressed some thirty years earlier by the Halle professor Friedrich Hoffmann: 'sic enim novi feminas, quae inter iocos cum marito a sola fortiori mammarum contrectatione loco iucunditatis perpetuum morbum et luctum reportarunt' (For thus I know women who, when frolicking with their husband, because of a single rather fierce manipulation, instead of pleasure had to carry with them permanent disease and sorrow).[85] After the principal character in Goethe's *Wilhelm Meisters Lehrjahre* (written in 1795–96) had passionately embraced the countess, that young woman felt absolutely certain that she was going to develop a breast cancer since a portrait medallion of her husband, which she was wearing at that moment, had painfully pressed her bosom, and no physician could talk her out of it.[86] Trauma of any type was believed either to disrupt the glandular ducts, releasing their contents into the interstitial mass, or to loosen their elasticity, with intraductal stagnation as a result.[84] It was generally thought, as a matter of course, that scirrhous tumours of traumatic origin would better lend themselves to treatment than similar growths proceeding from internal derangement of humours.

Surgeons were divided in their opinion as to the exact nature of the body juice which, from whatever cause, stagnated and coagulated within the corpus mammae. Galen's atrabiliary doctrine was far from forgotten, but had gradually acquired a more modern look in which black bile — a humour always a bit difficult to explain — and the ensuing 'melancholia' had taken on a new significance. As Boerhaave had pointed out, the four cardinal humours of the ancients were in fact only different parts of the blood. Aptly summarized by Lester King, Boerhaave taught that 'Galen's "yellow bile" was only the blood serum and not bile at all. The "phlegm" was only the altered serum into which the yellow bile changed by standing and the atrabile or "black bile" of Galen, was only a part of the "crassamentum" (red clot) which separated off and assumed a much darker colour'.[87] Two former Boerhaave students, Johannes de Gorter (1689–1762), a MD-surgeon who ultimately became physician to the imperial court in St. Petersburg, and Gerard van Swieten in Vienna, simply used the ancient term 'melancholia' for the black, 'earthlike' constituent of the blood.[88, 89] Because of its pitch-like stickiness this matter could easily choke the minor vessels, causing stasis and tumefaction. This would happen, explained de Gorter more fully, in cases of inflammation, when blood would contain a 'materia phlogistica', an initial stage of pus.

34

Should this fluid material come to a standstill in a gland, its thin components would gradually separate and drain off, leaving the thick constituents behind. Drying-in of the deposit would result in scirrhus.[90]

The old Galenic idea that scirrhus was a kind of inflammation[91] had been revived by Boerhaave, who in 1709 had advanced the theory that scirrhus should be regarded as the remains of an acute inflammation which had not ripened to the point of perforation, but had not completely resolved either.[92] Later in the century John Hunter taught that 'a species of suppuration' was taking place in the centre of a malignant tumour.[93] Hunter, however, unlike de Gorter, was a partisan of the lymph theory of cancer. His views on the disease were not particularly original.

The French school represented by Jean Astruc and others also adhered to Sylvius' lymphogenous theory; van Swieten in Vienna voiced the opinion that retention of curdled milk was the basic pathology underlying the scirrhus,[94] a view shared by the famous *Encyclopédie* first edited by Diderot and d'Alembert.[95] The lymphogenous theory seemed to be endorsed by experiments carried out by François Gigot de Lapeyronie (1667–1747), surgeon to King Louis XV and founder of the Académie de Chirurgie. As described by François Quesnay (1694–1774), permanent secretary of the Royal Academy of Surgery in Paris, small slices of tumour were cut from a diseased breast after amputation and thrown into boiling water. They became hard and transparent. Thereupon some fluid, expressed from the centre of the tumour, was heated: it coagulated while acquiring a pale shade and a rather firm consistency, very much like the heated tissue. Moreover, it spread a fetid odour which put an end to any doubt that the humour which engorged the tissue of the tumour was veritable lymph already strongly corrupted.[96]

More complex were theories which were being developed in the course of the century and which, apart from blood or lymph, also included 'nourishing juices' and still other substances in their aetiological considerations. Thus, later in his life, the rich nerve supply of the breast gave Boerhaave (1744) the idea that 'liquor nervorum', the juice he believed to pass through tiny channels thought to exist in the nerves, might give rise to scirrhous growth when it mixed with fluid discharged by the mammary gland proper.[83]

If there existed a number of different views on the development of scirrhus, there was no unanimity either as to how scirrhus, once established, could merge into cancer. Many adhered to the seventeenth-century notion that a particular 'acrimony' brought about the cancerous transformation. According to current opinion, such 'acrimony' could be a local product of coagulating fluids in decay within the mammary gland, or – which was regarded as less likely – might proceed from a wrong composition of body juices in general, or enter the blood from the outer world by way of spiced food. On the nature of the 'acrimony' most authors did not care to express themselves clearly. That such 'sharpness' was very 'sharp' indeed was obvious from the corroding juice discharged by ulcerous cancer. Van Swieten claimed that a linen cloth, used to cover such a defect, was once found to have been eaten away as if it were corroded by 'aqua fortis'.[89] Le Dran reported that he had felt a burning sensation in his face for some hours, while his garment became permanently discoloured in parts after an operation during which he had been splashed by cancer juice.[97]

A theory from the days of Sylvius held that, chemically speaking, the 'acrimony' would be acid. The Amsterdam surgeon, Anton Schrage (1765–1820), found support for this belief when he experienced a distinctly acid sensation upon placing a slice of diseased mammary tissue on his tongue. Not yet entirely satisfied, he slowly heated some blood of the same patient to test its reaction. During this experiment his face was struck by such acid fumes that, observing a laboratory tip once given by Boerhaave, he deemed it prudent to expose his head to the vapour of hot urine, by way of counteraction. After this experience the industrious investigator was quite satisfied that an acid factor was present in cancer patients, both in the tumour itself and in the circulating blood.[98] Quesnay, on the other hand, felt than when 'acrimony' was not a product of fermentation but was derived from silent or incomplete putrefaction, it would chemically be alkalescent or alkaline.[96] Richard Guy in London found that tumour masses spread a fume with 'an alkaline smell' when boiled.[99] Jean Astruc denied the presence of any 'sharp' material since he did not find any difference in salt content between a removed cancerous breast and a piece of beef of the same weight.[100] The data produced by eighteenth-century biochemistry were clearly non-conclusive.

To move from the notions of 'sharp acid' or 'putrefying alkali' to the concept of a specific 'cancer poison' does not require a great stretch of imagination. In fact, quite a few medical and surgical authors from the eighteenth century appear to have accepted the existence of 'cancerous matter',[101, 102] 'virus carcinomateux',[97, 103] or 'cancer poison'.[85, 104] To quote the *Encyclopédie*: 'a virus particulier dont on ignore absolument l'action méchanique, communément' was believed to be directly responsible for the development of malignancy.[105] According to Bernard Peyrilhe (1735–1804), stagnant lymph — the proximate cause of cancer — could, by a process of putrefaction, turn into a 'matière ichoreuse' from which the true cancer virus proceeded. Peyrilhe gave this explanation in a prize-winning essay, written in response to the terse question: What is cancer?, posed by the Academy of Science, Arts and Letters in Lyons in 1773. Peyrilhe was not just an ordinary surgeon. He was on the teaching staff of the Paris school of surgery. The most prominent of its kind in the realm, the school had been elevated to the dignified status of Collège de Chirurgie in 1750. Its professors were the pick of Paris surgeons. In his treatise, he expressed his belief in the essential identity of scirrhus and cancer and showed himself a partisan of radical surgery. Peyrilhe also performed what seems to be the first animal experiment in the history of oncology by instilling fluid derived from a cancerous breast into an artificial wound in the back of a dog. The wound was closed by adhesive plaster strips. Within a few days a crater-shaped ulcer developed. He could not reach a definite conclusion, however, because the dog kept howling and was drowned by Peyrilhe's housekeeper, who was apparently neither an animal lover nor a firm believer in science.[106] Le Cat[80] and Astruc[84] belonged to a minority group by denying the actual existence of any such 'virus'.

Two well-known Amsterdam surgeons, Jan Grashuys (1699–?)[107] and David van Gesscher (1736–1810),[108] held an uncommon point of view by regarding breast cancer not as a malady taking place in the mammary gland proper, but as a disease of the 'celwijs weefsel' (cell-like tissue), which was made up of periglandular fat. Their solidistic concept deserves to be remembered for, about a century later, Virchow referred to Grashuys when he, in his turn, described cancer as a disease of connective tissue. The notion of 'tissue' appears to be in common use long before the foundation of histology by Bichat in 1800. In the first half of the century, Jean-Louis Petit, for instance, advised not to leave any cellular tissue behind when removing a cancerous breast.[109] The word 'cell' is not yet used in the sense of tissue-cell, however. It was employed to describe the macroscopic aspect of body fat. Camper in 1797 did look upon cancer as 'a wholly changed and destructed glandular mass', but it is not quite clear whether he discarded the influence of humours in its origin.[110] Menopause and all kinds of psychic influences are almost invariably cited in the medical literature of the eighteenth century as additional factors that might encourage the development of scirrhus of carcinoma. Some writers suggested in addition: family predisposition, childlessness, a sedetary life, bad dietary habits, late nights and the consumption of alcohol and coffee.

The importance attached to the cessation of menstruation is connected with the ancient Hippocratic belief that some sort of 'consensus' exists between the uterus and the breasts. Some authors explained the connection between breast cancer and meno-pause, or between breast cancer and menstrual disorders in younger women, by claiming that suppression of menstrual discharge – which was generally believed to be corrupted blood – would lead to corruption of humours already stagnant in the breast (e.g. le Dran).[97] Others, for example le Cat,[80] were satisfied with a vague notion of 'transplantation' or frankly admitted that they were unable to explain the connection. The importance attached at the time to the cessation of menstruation is also illustrated by the common advice to correct any irregular menstruation, by appropriate diets and drugs, when treating young cancer patients.

A causal connection was also widely believed to exist between haemorrhoids and mammary cancer, in that women who had suffered for a long time from bleeding piles – apparently a common ailment at that time – were also exposed to the danger of malignancy once bleeding had ceased, particularly if the blood had been dark.

It is surprising for modern eyes to see the great significance which surgeons in the seventeenth and eighteenth century attached to psychic determinants, not only to 'constitutional' melancholy, but also to deep sorrow or a bad fright. People with a melancholy temperament were predisposed to cancer since they were supposed to carry a relatively high level of material 'melancholia' in their blood.[111] Psychic factors are mentioned time and again in case reports. Hoffmann went so far as to contend that nine out of ten women with cancer had suffered from great grief.[85] In an elaborate psychosomatic explanation, le Cat surmised that sadness would bring on a constriction of the finest vessels with the consequence that fluids were driven into 'subaltern' vessels which were not really meant to contain any juices. Coagulation of the trapped humours would ensue.[80] The great Boerhaave also made allowance for the influence of dejectedness when he observed: 'cancer in femina plethorica facile curatur, difficillime in melancholica' (Cancer is easily treated in a plethoric woman; it is most difficult to treat, however, in a melancholic one).[83] Why Boerhaave should have thought that fullbloodedness was a favourable condition, I have been unable to ascertain. Lorenz Heister and quite a few other surgeons even advised against any operation in melancholic patients.[112]

Relatively few authors expressed opinions on the possibility of hereditary transmission. Hoffmann,[85] Joseph de Lassone (1717–88),[113] Le Dran[97] and others were willing to accept it: De Lassone assumed the existence of a 'virus héréditaire'. Peyrilhe, on the other hand, denied the existence of any hereditary factors.[106] Patients, however, gave evidence of firmly believing in family predisposition. A nineteen-year-old nun in Avignon, for instance, refused to be operated upon since her grandmother and a great-uncle had died from the disease. She assumed that cancer poison occurred in her family as a hereditary taint, so that an operation could not be of any possible help to her.[97]

Childlessness, on the other hand, was a condition which was put forward by many writers. Heister[102] and Hoffmann[85] observed that cancer affected unmarried and barren women in particular. The number of nuns who appear in French case-histories is indeed striking. The lay public was well aware of this predilection: a young woman once attributed her disease to not having had any children, for which state of affairs she blamed her husband, who was 'd'un certain âge'.[80]

Amidst the treatises on the nature and therapy of cancer which abound in eighteenth-century medical literature, we find the first clear evidence of the concept of metastasis. As early as 1735, de Gorter wrote on 'cancereuse stoffe' (cancerous matter) that, after entering into the circulating blood, may make 'een metastasis van de eene glandule op de andere' (a metastasis from one glandule to another).[114]

Whether the notion of haematogenic metastasis was introduced here for the first time in history, complete with its modern term, I cannot say. Quite a number of eighteenth-century medical writers, however, appear to be familiar with remote deposits which they clearly distinguished from direct outgrowth. According to le Dran, a corrupted humour could find its way from the diseased breast into the circulation of both blood and lymph and could thus give rise to metastases – his word – in the axillae, lungs, brain and bones. He based his pronouncement on post-mortem evidence. Curiously enough, he regarded axillary nodes as haematogenic deposits.[97] In Petit's opinion, however, glandular swellings in the armpit were only a confirmation of the lymphatic origin of cancer.[115] The possibility of liver involvement was not yet appreciated in the eighteenth century, although 'intestinal' dissemination was occasionally reported.

In 1769 and 1787, respectively, admirable anatomical studies on the lymphatics were published by William Hewson (1739–74) in London, a former pupil of Alexander Monro and John Hunter[116] and by Paolo Mascagni (1752–1815), professor of anatomy at Siena[117] (Fig. 15). Such studies, probably incited by the current interest in lymph as a fluid matrix of cancer, did much to elucidate the lymph drainage system of the breast. This, in turn, promoted the theory of lymphatic dissemination. Petrus Camper, for instance, first thought that cancerous poison spread from the diseased breast along muscles and nerves. After his discovery of the 'mossy glands', as he called them, alongside the internal mammary blood vessels, which he associated with the only too common experience of local recurrence, he was converted to the lymphogenous theory of transmission[110] (Fig. 16).

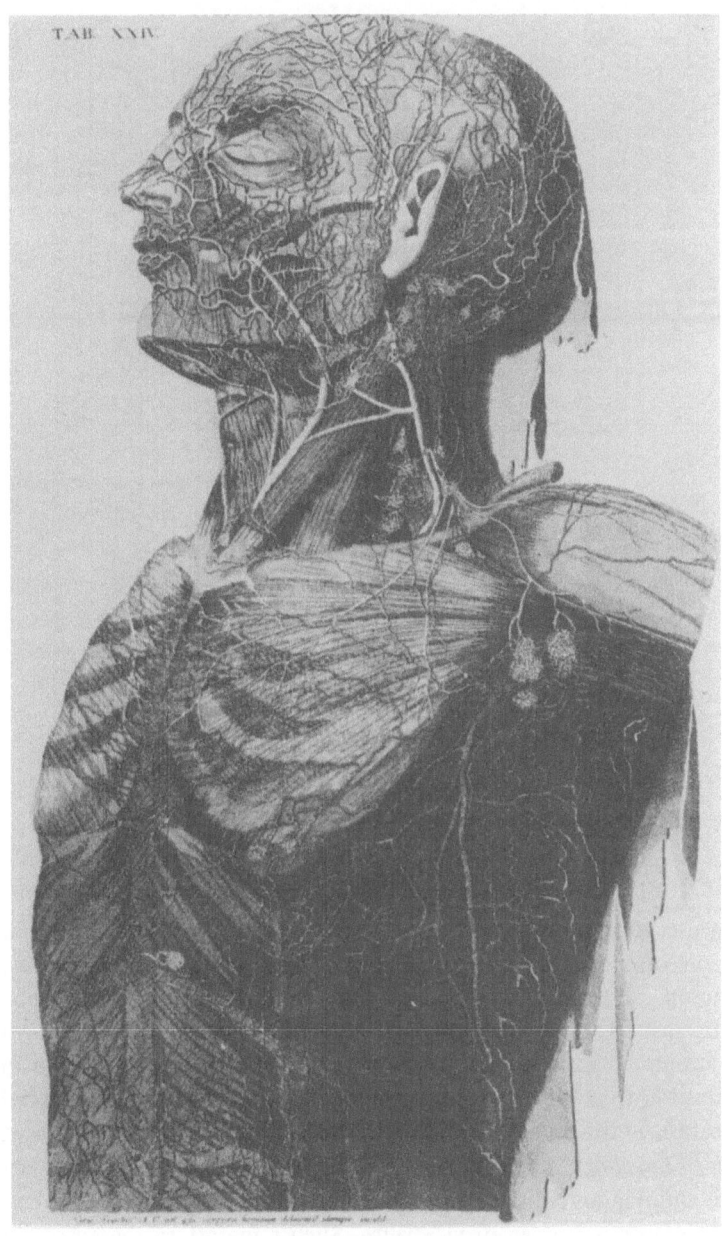

Fig. 15.   Pectoral lymph drainage according to Mascagni.

The concept of 'metastasis' still seems to have been somewhat alien to Giovanni-Battista Morgagni (1682–1771), the great eighteenth-century pathologist. In his famous book *De sedibus et causis morborum* (1761), which laid the foundation of morbid anatomy, Morgagni described a post-mortem case of pulmonary scirrhus fixed

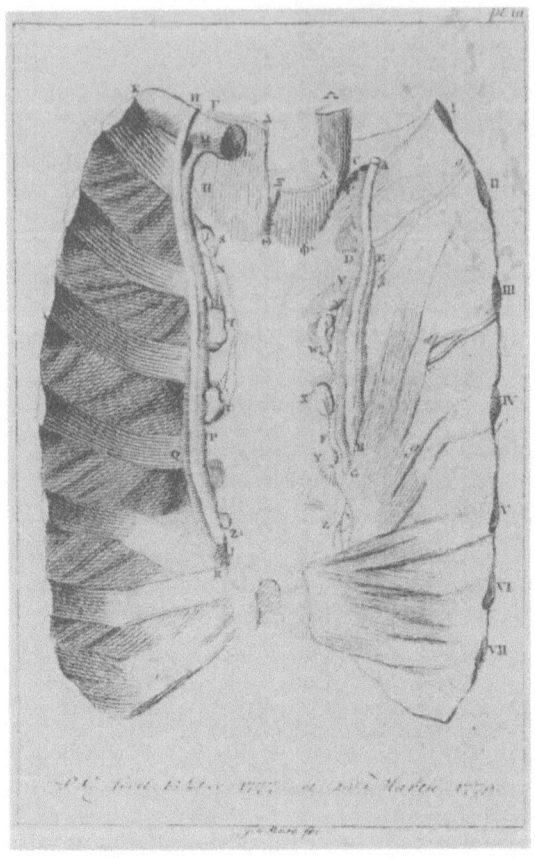

Fig. 16.   Internal mammary lymph nodes, described by P. Camper.

to the thoracic cage at the spot where ribs had come to be exposed some time after the amputation of a cancerous breast. On another occasion he noted the presence of a great lump of 'scirrhous tubercles' in the ipsilateral axilla. In both cases, however, he refrained from any comment. In the relevant chapters of Morgagni's book, the present author could find only one reference, and that, merely in a quotation from the literature, to a 'virus' which, by spreading over the sternum, was believed to have caused cancer in the heterolateral breast after amputation of the first breast.[77]

The French *Encyclopédie* carries a vast article under the reference 'metastase'. By that term the anonymous contributor meant, however, the spreading of a disease from the skin to some internal organ or vice versa. Such a metastasis, based on an ancient belief in some sort of mysterious 'remote sympathy' existing between different body structures, had of course, nothing to do with cancer. Progressive though it was in many aspects, the *Encyclopédie* was certainly not up to date in this respect.[118]

Within the theory that cancer results from a general derangement of body fluids, there is, of course, no room for such a notion as 'metastasis', since one and the same 'derangement' may well explain the presence of concomitant malignancies at different sites. Not all authors, however, felt the need for material explanations, such as those cited above. Le Cat thought it quite possible that breast cancer, even if it were of purely local origin, might, by causing general irritation, induce a 'cancerous disposition' in the whole body. Such a disposition might, in its turn, give rise to 'sympathetic cancer' elsewhere.[80]

Although the value of vital statistics slowly began to be recognized towards the end of the century, there are no reliable statistical data available on breast cancer. Le Dran wrote that it was a common disease.[97] Case histories, in so far as they pay attention to the 'duration' factor at all, only do so in patients who were remarkable for one reason or another. Thus, van Swieten cited the case of a patient who lived for two years with ulcerating breast cancer,[119] whereas Gerrit Jan van Wij, a surgeon in Arnhem (1748–1810), had an eighty-year-old patient who, with uncommon patience, suffered from an open cancer of more than thirty-years' duration, during which time the tumour gradually consumed the whole breast and affected the denuded ribs.[120] Van Wij quoted a surgeon by the name of J. de Man, who ascribed such dissimilarities to 'the difference that exists between bodies and bodies, and surely between cancer and cancer'.

Patients who died from their disease, did so from haemorrhage, at best, or from a general discomposition of the humours leading to emaciation and 'slow fever' whilst suffering horrible pain. The English poet Alexander Pope was referring to such pain − apparently endured with superhuman submission − when he ended his epitaph *On Mrs Corbet who died of a cancer in her breast* (about 1720?) with the words: 'The saint sustained it, but the woman died'.[121]

CHAPTER 5

Diagnosis and therapy
in the eighteenth century

Clinical diagnosis of breast cancer was easy in the many instances where patients presented themselves with an ulcerating, foul-smelling defect and complaining of intolerable pain. Van Swieten was amongst those who have left us with gruesome descriptions of such cases. If the lump had not yet penetrated the skin, the chief consideration was, of course, to distinguish between benign or malignant types of scirrhus and between scirrhus and scrofula — tuberculosis of the breast being by no means a rare occurrence at the time.[93] It was also important to decide whether the tumour had a local origin — trauma, inflammation, milk retention — or whether it resulted from an internal cause, such as a general corruption of humours, suppression of menstruation or melancholy. The occurrence of itch, burning and pain, especially of the lancinating type in a previously painless lump was an almost pathognomonic symptom announcing a turn towards malignancy. Some authors, for example van Swieten, mention anosmia as a typical symptom.[122]

Physical examination was limited to the affected breast and its immediate environment. Attention was paid to the colour of the skin, the presence or absence of swollen veins, the position of the nipple, the consistency of the tumour and the degree of irregularity of its surface, its fixation to the skin or to the thoracic wall. The examination was completed by a search for palpable nodes in the ipsilateral armpit, in the supraclavicular area and in the neck. If the tumour was smooth and mobile and menstruation was unimpaired, it was held to be of a benign nature. Camper, however, warned that it would never be possible on the basis of such findings to differentiate between benign and malignant growth.[110]

With regard to treatment, a great deal of attention was paid to conservative methods. Such methods seemed to have favourable results every now and then, and surgery often deterred patients as well as their surgeons. Conservative therapy was thought to be appropriate when scirrhous tumours did not yet show definite signs of degeneration or when patients were reluctant to undergo surgery, or in cases which, for technical reasons, were unsuitable for operation. Medical treatment was aimed at dilution of the stagnating, inspissated or coagulated juices, whatever their nature or provenance, and at restoration of their normal flow within the affected breast.[123] The pursuit of this aim required the use of local means, as well as of measures to improve the circulation of humours at large. Rational as this may sound, we find, amongst the many external drugs of vegetable, animal, or mineral origin, quite a few that had been in favour for centuries. In spite of a clear-cut definition of the aims to be pursued, therapy remained entirely empirical. There is little sense in enumerating the many remedies recommended by eighteenth-century therapeutists, but amongst the prescriptions for external use 'resolving' poultices and plasters in great variety, juice of the leaves of deadly nightshade, plantain or tobacco plants, arsenic paste in different compositions, and lead and mercury ointments can be found, as well as, in the case of ulceration, frogspawn, oil of baked frogs, rotten apples, fresh veal or even a pigeon or any other warm-blooded animal cut up alive[105] — though the latter medieval method was then rather obsolete. Fresh meat was thought by de Gorter and others to mitigate pain by absorbing the acrimonious discharge in cases of open cancer.[124] Fumigations with sulphur or exposure to acid vinegar fumes as recommended by Galen[89] also occur on the therapeutic list. Astruc confined himself to the use of simple compresses saturated with urine.[125] Richter recommended tar to counteract any evil smells.[126] More than once we hear the warning that external remedies, especially those of a corrosive nature, might aggravate rather than ameliorate the disease. Le Cat, for instance, was against the use of topical medicines at all.[80]

In the Age of Enlightenment it became unethical for members of the medical and surgical professions to make use of secret remedies. The public at large, however, valued them as ever before and quacks made a comfortable living by selling nostrums. These often contained arsenic or other traditional ingredients, such as crawfish pounded alive to a pulp-like mass.

Quite a new and progressive method of cancer treatment was by electricity, a phenomenon that commanded much interest at the time among scientists and lay public alike. The newly invented electric machines made it possible to generate electricity at any moment desired. Before long, doctors were treating, indiscriminately and purely by way of experiment, cases of paralysis, spasm, epilepsy, neuralgia, torticollis, tooth-ache, deafness, intermittent fever and insanity with the new medium. John Brisbane (d.1776?) in London and Andrew Duncan (1744–1828) in Edinburgh claimed favourable results in the treatment of breast cancer with this medium.[127] After their reports in 1772 and 1778, respectively, silence fell upon the subject. It is surprising to find that the electric eel, used in ancient times to combat head-ache among other things, was employed in the treatment of breast cancer as late as 1823![128]

External treatment was generally supported by internal therapy. The latter consisted of humidifying or diluting diets, or even a starvation cure, laxatives and medicines. Milk-diets occupied an important place in dietary treatment since milk was, just like mineral water, believed to palliate the sharp acrimony of the humours.[81, 85, 95, 97] Spiced food, of course, was forbidden. According to the *Encyclopédie*, broths prepared from chicken, frogs, or toads were useful to clear the blood of cancer virus.[105] Opium was given against pain. Amongst medicines administered orally, the juice of deadly hemlock (conium maculatum) and deadly nightshade (atropa belladonna) aroused great hopes for a while. The former drug was recommended by the Austrian court physician Anton von Stoerck (1731–1803) — he called the herb 'cicuta' — in 1760,[129] the latter became known after an elaborate publication (1754) by the Groningen professor of medicine and botany, Tiberius Lambergen.[130]

Before administering it to their patients, both physicians took the medicine themselves, in steadily increasing dosages, to test for possible harmful effects.

The Amsterdam surgeon, Schrage, who believed he had demonstrated the acid nature of cancer poison, consistently prescribed alkalescent or alkaline medication.[98] He was not altogether original, however, since Pierre Dionis (1710) had also recommended a diet rich in volatile, alkaline salts, together with alkaline medicines, though only after operation.[131] Camper (Fig. 17), who may indeed be regarded as a prominent eighteenth-century oncologist, denied that cancer could ever be cured by external or internal medication. He also rejected bloodletting, a procedure still favoured by some surgeons and physicians because it was believed to decrease the relative proportion of the potentially dangerous black and heavy components of the blood.[110]

In the literature consulted, most medical as well as surgical authors appear to favour operative treatment, at least in principle: 'with the knife we can go where the other can not reach', Hunter argued.[132] They enumerate, however, quite a number of contraindications. The most important of these were, for obvious reasons, internal factors, whenever they seemed to exist. A generally unfavourable physical condition and, as mentioned earlier, a melancholic character were also accepted reasons to abstain from surgery. Richter considered dyspnoea and stitches in the chest as contraindicant since they might denote induration of the lungs.[133] When pain was located alongside the sternum between the second and third ribs, it denoted that the internal mammary lymph glands were involved, according to Camper. Prognosis was, of course, absolutely unfavourable in such cases as well.[110] Further reasons to refrain from surgical intervention could be found in local circumstances: adherence, extension into the axilla, palpable nodes in the neck. If some surgeons were prepared to remove hardened axillary nodes together with the diseased breast, John Hunter warned that during the operation, often 'a chain is found to run far beyond out of our reach'. He held that 'we cannot be too nice in our examination, nor often too rough-handed in the operation'.[134] Much time was frequently lost in making efforts to dissolve the lump by conservative methods first, even when a positive diagnosis had been made and no contraindications seemed to forbid operation.[104] Quite a few surgeons, particularly in Amsterdam, had hardly any use at all for operative therapy, discouraged as they were by the disappointing results.[98]

All authors agreed that operative treatment should aim at complete removal of the morbid process. Should this not appear feasible, no operation was to be undertaken at all. 'The early period of the complaint is beyond all doubt, the most favourable period for extirpating it', wrote the British surgeon Henry Fearon (17?–1825?) in 1784. Unfortunately, 'patients can seldom be convinced that there is any necessity for an operation while the disease continues in a mild state...'.[135] Benjamin Bell (1749–1806), surgeon to the Royal Infirmary in Edinburgh and a former pupil of Monro, in 1784 advocated radical operation as soon as the diagnosis was made, even if the tumour was still very small. As little skin as possible should be excised, however.[136] Different modes of surgical approach existed at that time. Operations might vary from simple excision of the lump, as practised by William Cheselden in London and by René-Jacques Croissant de Garengot (1689–1759) in Paris, to an extensive mastectomy with excision of the pectoral fascia and removal of axillary nodes, as taught by Jean-

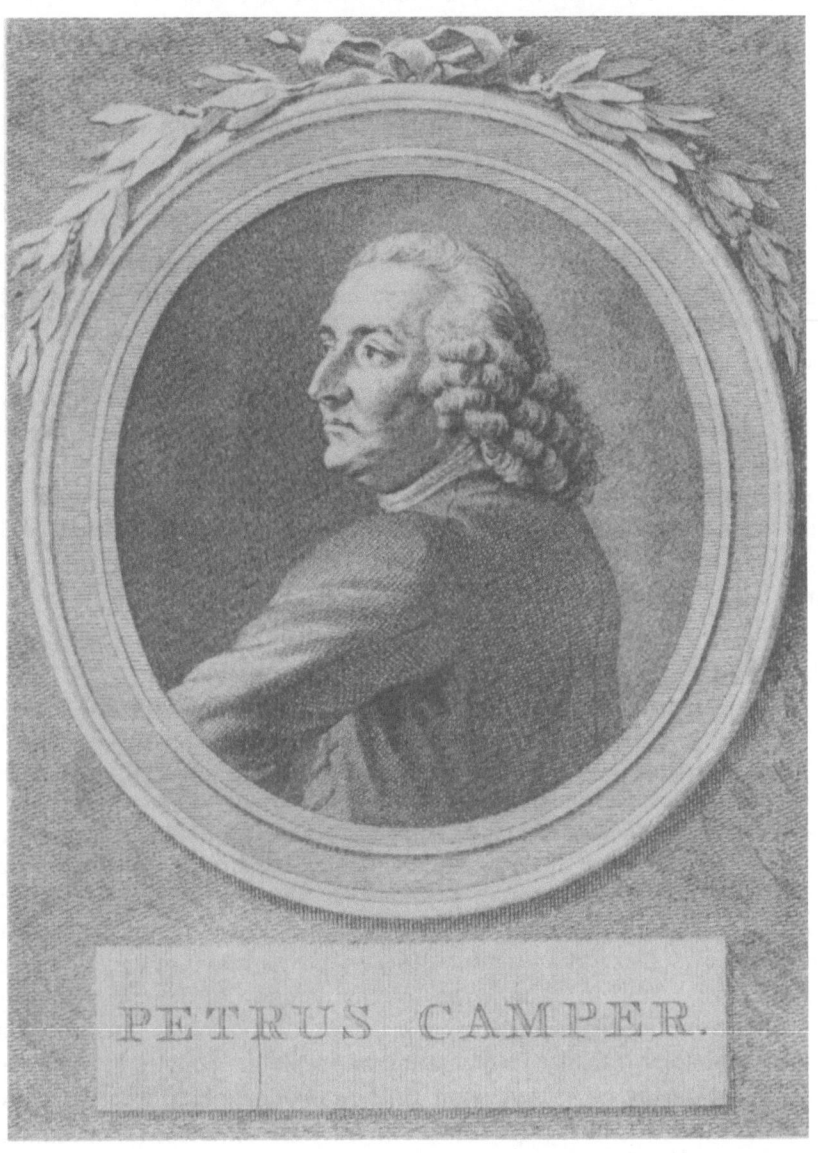

Fig. 17. P. Camper.

Louis Petit, who in 1731 had become the first Director of the French Academy of Surgery. Petit started by removing any axillary nodes.[137] Bernhard Perilhe, in his 1774 prize essay, even advocated the removal of the major pectoral muscle as well.[106] So it appears that the principles of what later would be known as Halsted's operation, were already formulated in the second half of the eighteenth century.

More and more surgeons aimed at wound healing by first intention, by saving an adequate skin area and uniting the edges by adhesive plaster or by stitches. Traditional ablation by a few rapid strokes of a razor remained common practice, however. This follows implicitly from a letter, written in 1751 by Madame d'Aguillon to Montesquieu, the well-known political philosopher, in which she casually informed her correspondent of the operation of Madame Marie-Louise de Bonnac. That lady's surgeon, Sauveur-François Morand (1697–1773) one of the most distinguished surgeons of his time, had told her beforehand, that he would not need more than one minute. 'Take four', the intrepid lady replied, 'and make a good job of it'.[138] In a handwritten, but unsigned case-history, presumably dating from 1772 and kept in the Public Records of the Dutch town of Middelburg, an anonymous surgeon – probably Samuel de Wind – noted that it had taken him two minutes to perform such an operation on Miss Elisabeth Carijn.[139] Such rapid mastectomies cannot have meant more than simple ablations.

Straightforward ablation without closure of the wound was also a method favoured by John Hunter as appears from a case-history which he presented to illustrate the importance of inspecting the operative specimen after removal 'to see if there are any corresponding appearances so as to lead to the supposition of a part being left'. When one day he did find such a suspected induration, he put the specimen back into the wound to find the corresponding part left behind, when he dressed the patient the next morning.[134]

To facilitate amputation of a breast at its base, Hendrik Ulhoorn designed a cutting clamp. This curious device, that might remind the modern reader of a huge cigar-cutter, is featured amongst the numerous fine illustrations of Lorenz Heister's text-book of surgery. Heister wrongly attributed the invention to a German surgeon by the name of Gerhard Tabor[76] (Fig. 18).

Preoperative measures consisted of bloodletting and purging and dietary rules along the lines followed in medical therapy. The ancient practice of allowing the wound to bleed a few ounces before applying a pressure bandage after the operation, was still followed. By now, however, this procedure was believed to prevent postoperative haemorrhage, inflammation and fever. Postoperative care was not confined to the wound. It was also aimed at prevention of recurrence by means of dietary measures as mentioned above, often to be observed for the duration of the patient's life. Some authors advised burning the extremities by means of thermocautery after the operation and encouraging their prolonged suppuration to enable the body to get rid of vitiated humours.[97] Treatment by cauterization of the tumour itself had become obsolete: Joseph de Lassone, personal physician to Queen Marie-Antoinette, condemned it as sheer 'barbarity'.[113] Great importance was attached to salves and other materials which could prevent the bandages from sticking to the wound. Without such pre-cautions, each change of dressing would prove extremely painful.

Operations were still carried out, if at all possible, in the patient's residence. The hospital still only cared for those whose conditions in life did not allow them to be ill at home.

As to the frequency with which breast operations were carried out, we have to be content with vague statements, like that of le Dran, who claimed to have carried out 'a great number' of operations, 'many' with success, or of Jacob van der Haar (1717–1799) in Bois-le-Duc who, in 1761, while discussing postoperative treatment casually

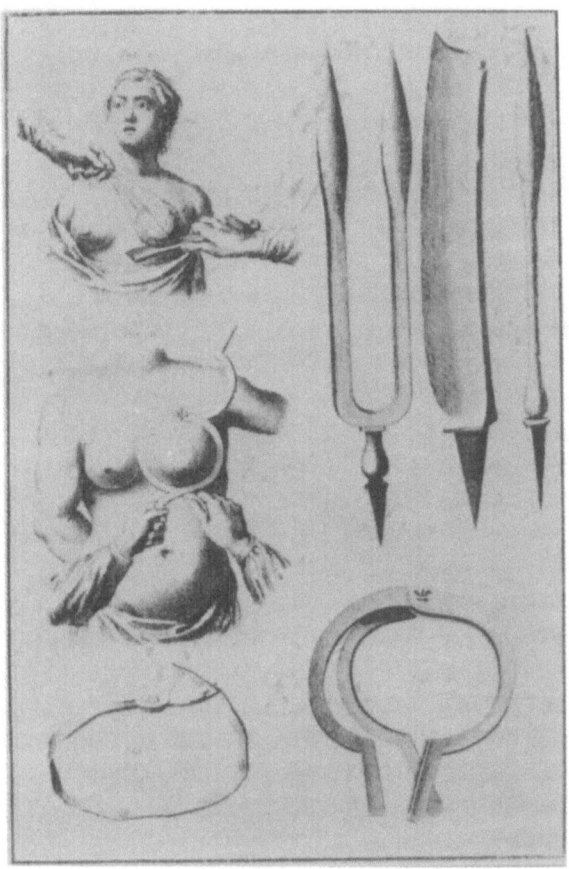

Fig. 18. An illustration from Diderot's and d'Alembert's *Encyclopédie*.

remarked that he had given Peruvian bark to fifty patients.[140] This would imply that he did at least two to three mastectomies a year.

There are a few statements from which it may appear that amputation was less frequently performed in the second half of the century. Thus, in 1747, Ulhoorn remarked that, in his day, the notion was dawning that there was no point in operating on even small tumours, when cancerous matter had already spread through the body. Ulhoorn did not make it clear, however, how such a dissemination could be ascertained. Thirty years ago, he added, this basic rule was not yet understood, and surgeons 'cut off everything they saw, as was the fashion'.[76] Camper, however, seemed to regret in 1757 that, in a densely populated town like Amsterdam, 'not six times a year a breast was amputated with reasonable chance of a cure'.[141] Amsterdam had about 200,000 inhabitants at the time.

Reliable postoperative survival rates are also lacking. Two conflicting reports, both from Edinburgh, were repeatedly quoted until far into the nineteenth century. The

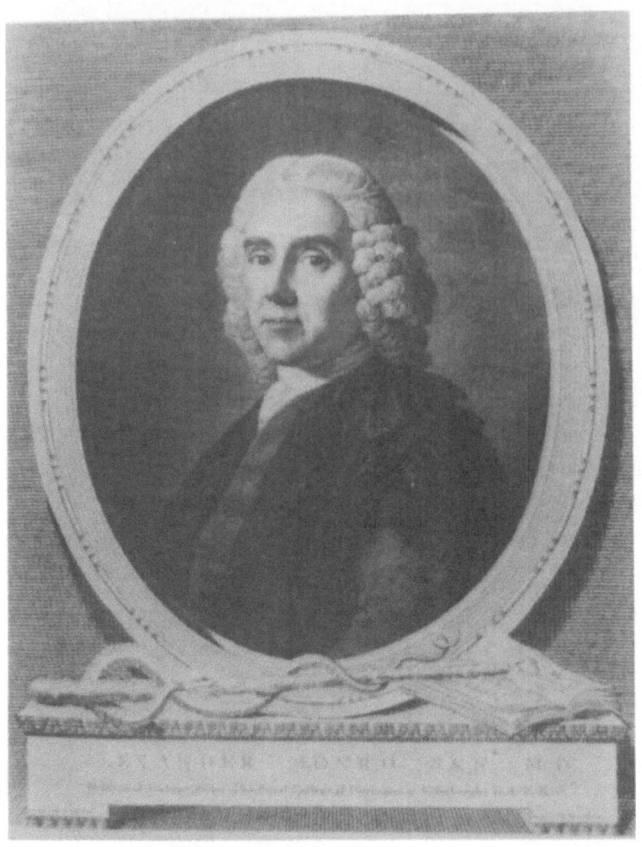

Fig. 19. Alexander Monro senior.

first one was written by Alexander Monro senior (1697–1767) (Fig. 19) and published by his sone in 1781. Out of sixty cases of cancer, Monro stated, only four patients appeared to be alive without signs of the disease after two years. Three of them had occult cancers in the breasts, the fourth had an ulcerated cancer of the lip. Monro held very ·pessimistic views with regard to cancer. The disease nearly always returns after the operation, not invariably to the part where it was taken away, but frequently in the neighbourhood or even at a considerable distance. Operative treatment should only be undertaken in a young and healthy woman with an occult cancer evoked by a bruise or some other external cause. In all other cases, an operation should only be proceeded to at the earnest request of the patient who had had the danger of relapse clearly explained to her.[142] Monro was an influential author. His rejection of mastectomy certainly contributed to the conservative attitude adopted by many surgeons towards the end of the century. A former Monro student, James Hill, could, on the other hand, boast of 76 cases from a total of 88, that were perfectly cured by operation.[143] Richter might well wonder, whether the two Scots had been treating the same disease.[144]

The eighteenth century saw the beginning of a continued follow-up of patients who had been operated upon or otherwise treated: Le Dran, Lambergen and Camper may be cited amongst those who kept in touch with at least some of their patients for years.

Surgical literature of the eighteenth century abounds with case reports; a mastectomy was apparently still of sufficient interest to warrant a publication. These reports gradually became more extensive and more detailed, with the result that more and more patients emerge from them as individual women. It is not unusual to find them referred to by name.

Heister expressed his view on the cancer patient and her surgeon as follows: 'Many females can stand the operation with the greatest courage and without hardly moaning at all. Others, however, make such a clamour that they may dishearten even the most undaunted surgeon and hinder the operation. To perform the operation, the surgeon should therefore be steadfast and not allow himself to become disconcerted by the cries of the patient'.[76] In the last sentence, Heister was paraphrasing a frequently cited piece of advice from the Roman Aulus Cornelius Celsus.[13] In doing so, he unwittingly showed that, even after eighteen centuries, operative surgery had not become easier, either for the patient or for the surgeon.

One of the typical aspects of the Age of Enlightenment was a gradual awakening to the recognition that the socially strong should be responsible for the weak. The weak in society certainly included the indigent cancer patient. In 1740, the first hospital exclusively for such patients was founded in Reims by Jean Godinot, a canon of the cathedral. It contained twelve beds.[68] Private charity also enabled the opening of a free cancer ward in the Middlesex Hospital in London in 1792 (Fig. 20). Here the

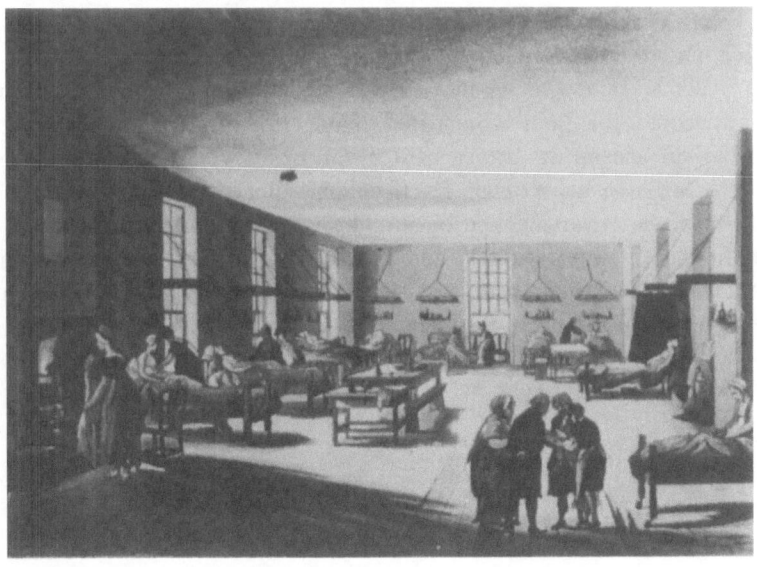

Fig. 20. Middlesex Hospital, London.

49

initiative came from the surgeon John Howard (?–1810 or 11). The arguments with which he had persuaded the Board of Directors of the Middlesex Hospital to reserve an unoccupied ward for the exclusive care of cancer patients, were of two kinds. Being looked after in a hospital would lighten the burden of those who were suffering from the disease and, secondly, cancer patients who stayed for an unlimited time would give physicians an opportunity to study 'the natural history' of the disease. A better knowledge of the natural history might improve treatment. Howard also proposed the establishment of an out-patient service.

A substantial endowment from Howard's friend Samuel Whitbread enabled the plan to be realized. During the nineteenth century, the Middlesex 'Cancer Charity' received important financial support from several other private persons, which contributed to the gradual development of that institution from a kind of nursing home to a modern cancer institute, consisting of a hospital with all sorts of therapeutic facilities and a research center all in one.[145] In the following chapters we will have the opportunity of referring to several important scientific contributions made by Middlesex men.

Ten years after the foundation of the Middlesex Hospital Cancer Charity, a number of prominent London physicians and surgeons established a Society for Investigating the Nature and Cure of Cancer. It issued a remarkable questionnaire, consisting of thirteen well-formulated questions regarding the diagnosis, pathogenesis and heredity of cancer. It appears that no answers were received. Four years later, in 1806, the enquiry was repeated with a similar result. Thereupon the Society seems to have declined.[145]

In the eighteenth century, yet another feature of the Enlightenment appeared in the history of cancer, namely public instruction. Newspapers became interested in the subject and advised their readers of remarkable cures, performed by surgeons and empirics alike. An example of the first, quoted from the *Hamburgischer Correspondent* of 1726, recounted how nimble-fingered surgeons in Genova cured breast cancer within two weeks by operation. A nice specimen of unorthodox medicine is provided by the happy cure of a poor woman near Hungerford in England, who had been suffering from an ulcerating breast cancer for many years. A certain gentleman prescribed live toads to be applied. These animals diligently sucked out the cancer poison until they were overwhelmed by it and died under convulsions. At the cost of 120 toads, the patient was definitely cured.[146] In view of what regular medicine had to offer by way of external therapeutics, one can hardly reproach the eighteenth-century newspapers for not being sufficiently critical!

CHAPTER 6

Europe during Napoleon and after

The revolution, which towards the end of the eighteenth century swept away the 'ancien régime' in France, also brought about a complete change in medical and surgical education. The old 'Facultés de Médecine' and the Paris 'Collège de Chirurgie' dating from 1750 were abolished. 'Ecoles de Santé', established in Paris, Montpellier and Strasbourg, were to take over and teach an integrated course, which meant that henceforth surgery was on a par with internal medicine. Great importance was attached to the observation and treatment of patients: 'Peu lire, beaucoup voir et beaucoup faire', was the maxim adopted by Antoine-François Fourcroy (1755–1809), one of the authors of the reformation.

The clinical teaching Paris took place, as of old, in the hospitals: in the Hôtel-Dieu, by far the largest with its 1500 beds, in La Charité and in a few others. For some time before the revolution, the Paris hospitals had been of very great significance for the teaching of surgery in particular. From 1780 on, Pierre-Joseph Desault (1744–95), who was chief surgeon at Hôtel-Dieu ever since 1784, has been making important alterations in the educational program for students of surgery. The facilities for clinic-attendance and operations were extended. Students were given their own responsibilities with respect to patient care, among other things, that of keeping clinical records.[147] In clinical teaching, much emphasis was placed on the relationship between clinical signs and post-mortem findings: this ushered in a flourishing of pathological anatomy. Ancient humoralism was gradually being defeated by the morphological approach and had to abandon the field of serious science.

The educational reforms of Desault had considerable consequences for the functioning of the hospital. Previously, in accordance with the Christian ideal of the Middle Ages, it had mainly been a place where indigent patients could find shelter, food and elementary care, free of charge, but henceforth it became a centre for the study of disease and the training of doctors. A place, moreover, where seriously ill patients could receive medical treatment according to the latest views.

Napoleon's wars contributed greatly not only to the development of operative surgery, but also to medicine, since many famous internists like Laennec, Broussais, Récamier and Cruveilhier, who were foremost in French medicine in the post-Napoleonic era, had been military surgeons in their younger years. The eminently practical attitude of these former army doctors perhaps explains why pathological anatomy came to occupy such an important place in the French clinic. The

51

introduction of percussion and auscultation also meant a very important step forward in the development of French clinical medicine.

Prominent surgeons, among others Alfredo-Armand-Louis-Marie Velpeau (1795–1867), a farrier's son who himself had been working as a farrier until his seventeenth year, for their part liked to regard surgery as 'manual medicine' and labeled their textbooks of surgery *Médecine opératoire*.[148]

After Napoleon's final downfall in 1815, Paris once again became a centre of medicine and surgery which attracted students from all over Europe and even from the United States of America.

In Germany, quite a different development had been taking place in the same period. There, the approach of medicine was philosophical rather than by means of the dissecting knife. Friedrich Schelling (1775–1854) taught in his natural philosophy that the entire cosmos was one immense, living being and that material nature, in view of the oneness of all, was not basically different from the mind. Thus it would be possible for the scrutinizing human mind to penetrate nature and arrive at true knowledge by a process of dynamic contemplation. It may be imagined that scientific medicine did not benefit much from such an approach.

Since no social revolutions, wars on her own territory, or new philosophy had occurred in Great-Britain, medicine in the British Isles continued for some time to bear the hall-mark of the eighteenth century. The main centres were London, Edinburgh, Glasgow and Dublin. In London, medical schools were connected with St. Bartholomew's, St. Thomas', Westminster, Guy's, St. George's, The London Hospital and the Middlesex. There were also private anatomy schools in that city, established in the eighteenth century for the study of surgery in particular. Some of these, like the one operated by William Hunter in Great Windmill Street, had attained a good reputation. The anatomy schools were abolished after 1824.[149]

Edinburgh was the scene of the mastectomy described by Dr. John Brown (1819–62) in his classic story *Rab and his friends* (1863). This narrative was based on an actual occurrence. The operation took place in 1830, when the author was clinical clerk at the Minto Hospital in the Scottish capital. The surgeon was James Syme (1799–1870), one of the most accomplished surgeons in the whole of Europe. His daughter married Joseph Lister. The moving scene was enacted in a semi-circular, wooden amphitheatre, similar to the one in the old St. Thomas' Hospital in London, which now serves as a museum. The gallery was filled with students. Amongst the onlookers was the patient's husband James and his dog Rab.

Ailie stepped up on a seat, and laid herself on the table, as her friend the surgeon told her; arranged herself, gave a rapid look at James, shut her eyes, tested herself on me, and took my hand. The operation was at once begun; it was necessarily slow; and chloroform — one of God's best gifts to his suffering children — was then unknown. The surgeon did his work. The pale face showed its pain, but was still and silent. Rab's soul was working within him; he saw that something strange was going on, — blood flowing from his mistress, and she suffering; his ragged ear was up, and importunate; he growled and gave now and then a sharp impatient yelp; he would have liked to have done something to that man. But James had him firm, and gave him a glower from time to time and an intimation of a possible kick; — all the better for James, it kept his eye and his mind off Ailie.

It is over: she is dressed, steps gently and decently down from the table, looks for James, then, turning to the surgeon and the students, she curtsies, — and in a low, clear voice, begs their pardon if she has behaved ill. The students — all of us — wept like children; the surgeon wrapped her up carefully, — and, resting on James and me, Ailie went to her room, Rab following. We put her to bed.[150]

Four days after the operation a septic infection developed of which the patient subsequently died. Ailie Noble showed an admirable self-restraint during the operation by being still and silent, but the procedure must have been extremely painful in the days before anaesthesia. The British novelist and essayist, Edward Morgan Forster (1879–1970), once published a letter, written by his great-aunt Miss Marianne Thornton in 1832, in which she recalled the 'awful screams' of Harriet Melville while she was operated on by Benjamin Brodie (1783–1862), whose name is still associated with chronic abscess of the tibia and with serocystic disease of the breast. Poor Harriet's screams 'sent Lucy into hysterics and drove Melville out of the house, as they penetrated even into his room. I never believed before, that the human voice had such strength'.[151] The English novelist Fanny Burney, whose operation we will touch upon presently, also marvelled at the strength of the voice of a woman, who had to suffer mastectomy.

The new clinical approach and the study of pathological anatomy by which the French school of medicine was rightly earning world fame in the first decades of the nineteenth century had, for the time being, no impact on the management of breast cancer. The relevant chapters in the textbook, which appeared in eleven volumes between 1818 and 1826, by Alexis Boyer (1757–1833), surgeon to La Charité, were mainly conceived in the spirit of the preceding century.[152] Of course, the greater part of Boyer's life took place in that age. The affliction was said to occur predominantly in women with a bilious constitution and a dejected, melancholy character, in whom sensibility and irritability were strongly developed.[153] Sensibility and irritability were concepts that, under the influence of the pathophysiological theories conceived by professor William Cullen (1712–92) in Edinburgh and by his compatriot John Brown (1735–88), for some time occupied an important place in medical thinking. The nervous system held a central place in their theories; health depended on adequate responses of the organism to the internal and external stimuli to which it is constantly being exposed. Such theories had, however, little impact on cancerology.

Boyer imputed the proximate cause of cancer to 'une diathèse particulière dont le principe est tout à fait inconnu'.[154] As the Swiss medical historian Erwin Ackerknecht recently pointed out, the word 'diathesis' acquired its present meaning of predisposition to certain disease only in the eighteenth century. It became a concept of central importance round about the turn of the century, particularly in Paris, the new capital of pathological anatomy. The abandonment of the theory of the humours and the introduction of solidism and localism had left medicine without a general coherent theory which could conveniently explain the material cause of disease. The new concept of predisposition, bearing the old name of 'diathesis', seemed, at first, to compensate for the loss.[155] There was no consensus, however, on the question whether diathesis should be looked upon as a pathologic or a premorbid condition. Many authors tried to explain predisposition by a particular condition of the blood, others thought it better not to express opinions on its exact nature.

Boyer's efficient causes, external as well as internal, are similar to those we met when we analysed oncological conceptions in the Age of Enlightenment. He may have been the first, however, to describe the clinical sign of 'peau d'orange' although he did not use the name.[156] Lymph nodes became only secondarily involved, subject to the condition that they are in direct communication with the diseased part by way of 'vaisseaux absorbans'.[157]

His therapy was also traditional. He displayed a profound pessimism as to the results of any method of treatment. He had personally operated on more than a hundred cases of cancer, in the breast and elsewhere, but only four or five of them had been radically cured. The first requisite for success is to operate at a very early stage. When that stage has passed, the surgeon should only proceed to operation at the urgent request of the patient after having informed her of the risk of recurrence.[158] The same warning had also been uttered by Monro, 50-odd years earlier.

A concept of diathesis, clearly different from Boyer's, was adopted by Philibert-Joseph Roux (1780–1854), a surgeon who, like Boyer, was attached to La Charité hospital. He attributed cancer to an external cause and regarded the affliction as initially a local process. By 'diathesis', he understood the general condition of the body, with cachexia as the extreme form, once the disease had spread. In his view, 'diathesis' was a result rather than a cause. Spreading would occur under 'sympathetic influence'; Roux did not believe in the existence of a cancer virus that might attack other organs via the cirulating blood.[159] 'Sympathy' was a mysterious association that might exist between two or more separate organs.

The age-old controversial question relating to the contagiousness of cancer — it had been revived by The London Society for Investigating the Nature and Cure of Cancer in 1802 — was definitely settled by experimental evidence which became available round about 1820. Two prominent dermatologists, Jean-Louis Alibert (1766–1837) and Laurent-Theodore Biett (1781–1840) had inoculated themselves with ichorous matter from cancer sores without contracting the disease. The surgeon Guillaume Dupuytren (1778–1834) used more caution in his relevant experiments when he fed his dogs with cancerous meat. The animals' health did not suffer either.[160]

The travel journals and diaries of foreign students who visited the French capital in the first half of the nineteenth century give precious information on how the famous Paris surgeons actually treated their patients. Roux, whom we have just mentioned, was one of the foremost surgeons of his time and his clinical demonstrations and his operations in La Charité attracted much interest. One day in 1815 there was, among his audience, a young English surgeon by the name of John Green Crosse (1790–1850). With respect to a breast operation performed by Roux, he inserted the following in his diary: 'They had neglected to shave ye axilla and before ye gland could be carried out it was obliged to be done when ye operation was thus far advanced'. The reader should keep in mind, that surgical anaesthesia had not yet been introduced at that time. At the first dressing, four days later. Crosse recorded: 'There was a horrible fetor and black dark discharge, with the surface of the wound dark and sloughing, edges of ye wound dry and elevated and indolent looking'.[161]

Three years later, the Leyden surgeon H.J. Logger described a mastectomy he had seen performed by Boyer. This extirpation of an open cancer from the left breast of a woman lasted ten minutes. The degeneration was removed by two horizontal half-moon shaped incisions of considerable extension since the whole mammary gland was diseased. Thereupon several more considerable indurations had to be detached from the surface of the thoracic wound, and finally also a few more indurations from the armpit at the same side. Boyer explained at length the reason for his different actions, and had the woman wait in the meantime. Five ligatures were applied to the breast, one in the axilla. The very large wound surface was covered with charpie; the sides of the wound were approximated over it as much as possible by means of adhesive plaster, and thereupon longuettes, compresses and a bandage were applied. The axilla was filled with charpie and covered with compresses.

The Leyden surgeon, who had himself been in practice for many years, did not always approve of what he had seen in Paris. When he saw Antoine Dubois perform a mastectomy, for instance, he was surprised to find that the surgeon did not search for any other indurations and that he departed, before all the bleeding vessels were tied, leaving it to his assistant to complete the operation.[162] Professor Dubois (1756–1837) was much in demand, as an obstetrician as well as a surgeon. In 1811, he presided over the mastectomy which the English novelist Fanny Burney (Fig. 21) had to undergo because of a lump that had troubled her for nearly a year. Some nine months after-wards, Fanny Burney, who had been living with her French husband in Paris since 1802, gave a vivid account of her dreadful experience in a letter to her sister in England.[163] At first, the tumour had not given her much concern, she wrote, although it was becoming increasingly painful. Her husband, however, had insisted that she seek medical advice and after a delay of several months, Antoine Dubois was sent for. In those days, physicians and surgeons did not have regular consulting hours. Those who were attached to a hospital had free clinics for the indigent and other patients were seen in their own homes. Dubois tried to reassure the patient, but he informed her husband at the same time of the gravity of the disease. He prescribed some medicine and excused himself, leaving the couple in a state of utmost anxiety. Since Dubois was in charge of the impending confinement of the Empress Marie-Louise, he was somewhat preoccupied.

Dominique-Jean Larrey (1776–1842), Napoleon's famous army surgeon, was now called in. Mrs. Burney, who wrote of him with great appreciation described him as a man 'with an ignorance of the world and its usages that induces a naivete that leads those who do not see him thoroughly to think him not alone simple but weak'. Logger, who visited Larrey's clinic in the Hôpital de la Garde in 1818, also depicts him as a modest man 'who distinguished himself most favorably from most of the other medical despots'. Larrey's unassuming manner may explain why, after still more consultations and delay, when he ultimately came to perform the mastectomy, Dubois acted as commander in chief, telling Larrey where and what to cut. The operation took place in the patient's bedroom. Fanny Burney's description of the preparations, such as hiring women who could take care of her after the operation – trained nurses did not

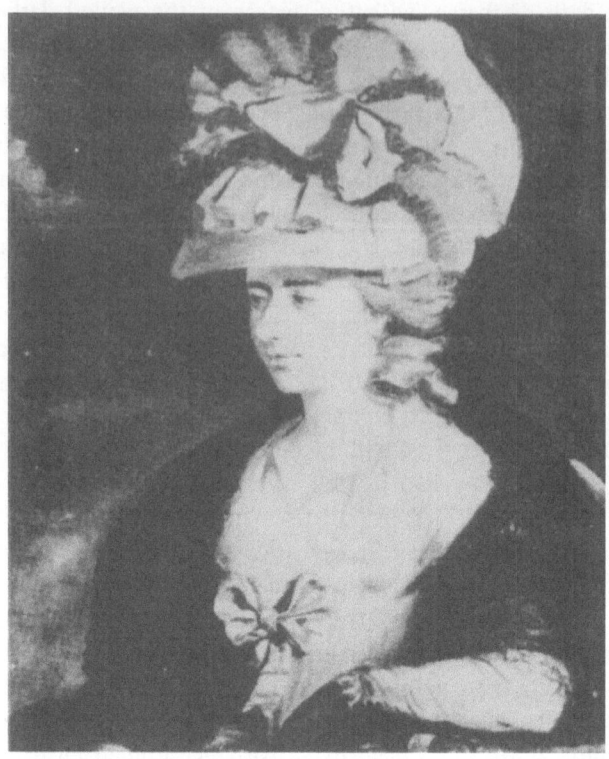

Fig. 21.   Fanny Burney.

yet exist — and making a will, the anxiousness caused by a delay of three whole weeks after she had given her consent, the excruciating agony of the intervention itself together form a moving, subjective account of what patients had to endure in the days of pre-anaesthetic surgery. It may have been common practice to postpone the scheduled operation for an unspecified time, meanwhile leaving the patient uncertain as to the precise date. In 1751, Madame de Bonnac was taken by surprise in the same way by her surgeon Morand.[138] The exact mode of the operation does not, of course, become clear from Mrs. Burney's account, but it seems to have been a traditional mastectomy, without additional removal of axillary nodes. The fact that she did not contract a sepsis may be attributed to her being operated upon in her own house, rather than in a hospital, the latter being a reservoir of infection. Since she survived her operation for about thirty years, we may have some doubt as to the malignant character of her affliction.

It is clear that the ever-present danger of septic infection and the lack of anaesthesia prohibited the development of better methods of operative surgery than those that had been in use for a thousand years. It is easy to understand, therefore, why quite different approaches were tried. In Great Britain, a certain Samuel Young divulged a method of treating tumours of the breast by continued compression. Before long, compression was considered the treatment of choice for breast cancer in England. In

France, the method was propagated by Joseph-Claude-Anthelme Récamier (1774–1856), physician to the Hôtel-Dieu in Paris. In his *Recherches sur le traitement du cancer par la compression méthodique simple ou combinée* (Paris, 1829), he reported on his results in one hundred cases. Thirty patients had recovered completely by compression alone, twenty-one had shown considerable improvement, fifteen of whom had been treated by compression followed by operation, and six by compression in combination with cauterisation. Twelve patients did not respond favourably.

After initial enthusiasm, critical voices were heard. A serious objection was that compression was difficult to apply evenly without leading to pain or even causing necrosis. Dr. Neil Arnott (1788–1874) of London therefore devised an apparatus in which pressure was exerted on the breast by means of an air-cushion (Fig. 22). Still more serious was the objection raised by such authorities as Alfred Velpeau (1835) and Hermann Lebert (1851), two prominent mid-century oncologists to whom we will presently turn our attention. They concluded that no definite cure of cancer had ever been obtained by the method and that alleged cures had actually no bearing on cancer cases. Compression treatment thereupon fell into disuse.[164]

In the early years of the nineteenth century, less progress was made regarding the treatment of tumours than in the knowledge of their minute structure. The latter development was initiated by Marie-François-Xavier Bichat (1771–1802), a pupil of Desault and the founder of histology. In his *Anatomie générale appliquée à la physiologie et à la médecine*, which appeared for the first time in 1801, he wrote that the different kinds of cancer consist more or less distinctly of connective tissue. Such tissue is the general base for the nourishing parenchyma. 'Tous les tumeurs sont cellulaires, c'est leur caractère commun', he emphasised.[165] Once again, 'cells' are not

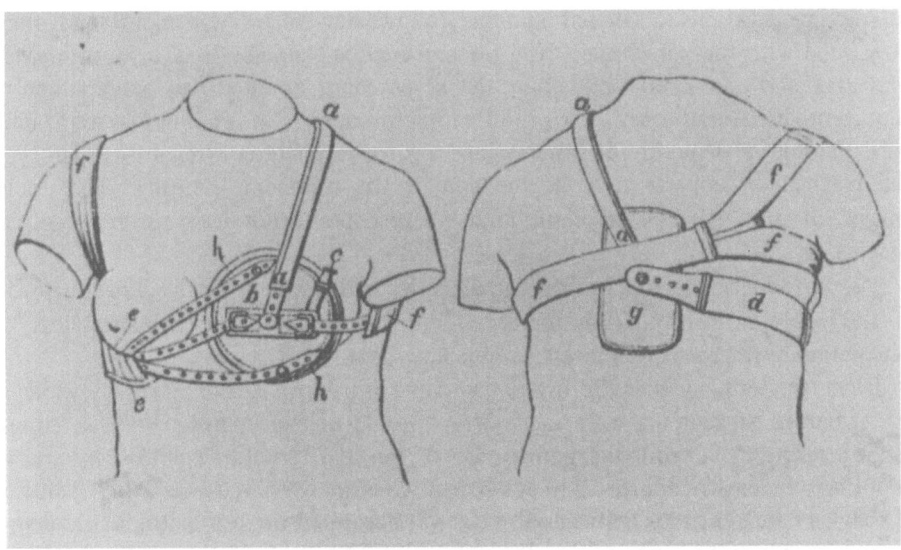

Fig. 22. Compression apparatus, designed by N. Arnott and described by W.H. Walshe.

to be understood in the modern sense, but as the interstices between the fibres that are just visible to the naked eye. Tumours only differed from one another by the nutritive elements that were deposited within these spaces. The 1830 edition was supplemented by an article by the anatomist-surgeon Pierre-Augustin Béclard (1785–1825), entitled 'Tissus accidentels'. This essay contains short, but excellent macroscopic descriptions of scirrhus ('il crie sous le scalpel') and of cancer. Béclard recognised only one 'cancerous tissue', the encephaloid matter that went under so many different names.[166] Bichat and Béclard did not make use of the microscope.

Bichat and his school laid the foundation of the solidistic concept of cancer that would become predominant in the nineteenth century. Amongst Bichat's pupils, René-Théophile-Hyacinthe Laennec (1781–1826) in particular is worthy of mention. Laennec is generally remembered for his invention of the stethoscope. In the history of oncology he achieved merit by devising a classification of tumours based, not on phenomenological aspects, as was previously customary, but on scientific principles. Thus, he distinguished between homologous tumours, that have an analogy in the body, and heterologous growths which, like the tubercle or scirrhus, do not bear any resemblance to normal tissue. In this view, scirrhus is not a pre-cancerous condition, but a particular kind of cancer. In contrast to the hard variety of cancer, which is represented by scirrhus, there is also a soft variety. Since its aspect is reminiscent of brain matter, Laennec named it 'encephaloid'.[167]

Another important representative of the Bichat school was Jean Cruveilhier (1791–1874), who became the first professor of pathological anatomy in Paris in 1836. Like Bichat, he did not attach much importance to the use of microscope. Cruveilhier defined cancer as a cancerous degeneration of normal tissue. In 1827, he stressed the pathognomic significance of white, creamy cancer juice, that, in varying quantity, always occurred in all types of cancer, especially the soft kind. There was a great deal of discussion about this cancer juice, mainly in French literature.[168]

The investigations of Bichat and his followers were, as was mentioned above, performed with the naked eye. After researchers like Malpighi, Hooke, Swammerdam, de Graaf and van Leeuwenhoek in the seventeenth century had made numerous important discoveries with their primitive microscopes – the capillary system, blood cells, the minute structure of some organs, protozoa, bacteria – scientific microscopy had reached an impasse towards the end of the eighteenth century. The unclear images of the uncorrected compound microscopes often lead to 'microscopical deceptions'.

The introduction of the achromatic objective by Hermanus van Deijl in Amsterdam in 1807 once again turned the microscope into a valuable scientific instrument.[169] A new period of microscopical investigations now began.

It was in Germany that the first important contributions to a better knowledge of the structure of tumours were made with the aid of the microscope. That country was liberating itself from the domination of speculative natural philosophy and was adopting a scientific approach to medicine, when in 1838 Matthias Jakob Schleiden (1804–81) and Theodor Schwann (1810–82) described the cell as the basic element of both plants and animals. As to the generation of cells, Schleiden and Schwann had postulated an amorphous formative substance, the blastema, from which nuclei

58

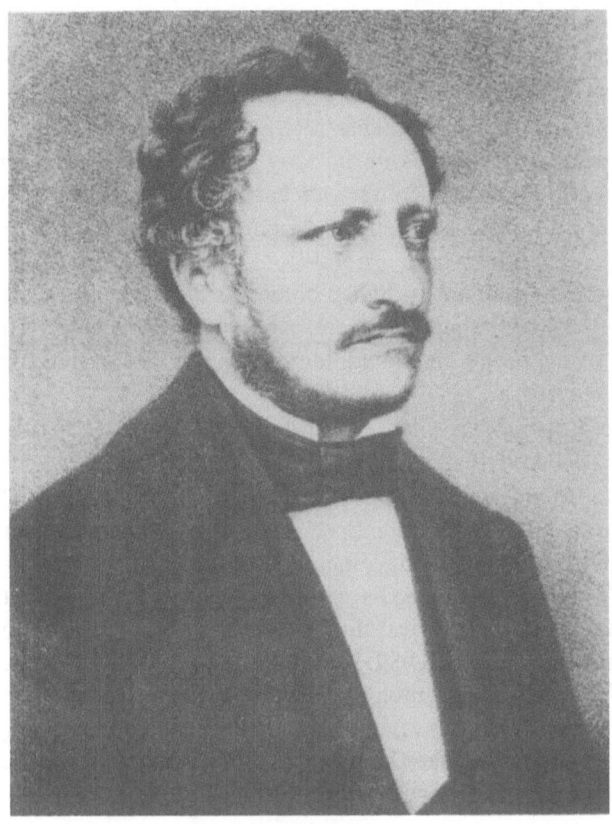

Fig. 23.   Johannes Müller.

would develop first, followed by cytoplasm surrounding them. Schwann likened this process to the precipitation of crystals in a saturated solution. The Greek word 'blastema', which means 'sprout', already occurs in Galen as one of the many descriptions used to define elevations, swelling or tumours.

Johannes Müller (1801–58) (Fig. 23), professor of anatomy and physiology in Berlin, may well be looked upon as the founder of cancer histology. Müller was an exceptionally versatile scientist who introduced modern experimental physiology in Germany. Microscopic anatomy was receiving much attention in his department, and it was probably no coincidence that, in the same year (1838), Theodor Schwann, who was working in Müller's department, described the animal cell and Müller himself published his treatise *Über den feinern Bau and die Formen der krankhaften Geschwülste*, which was to become a classic in the history of cancerology.[170] He established that pathologic growth consists of cells, just like any other tissue. In contrast to normal structures, however, the natural proportions had disappeared. The elements of form of cancerous growths are analogous to those of the normal elements of form of the body itself, or correspond with 'embryonic formations', as he called them, i.e. parts of tissue which are in a state of development. Most prominent amongst

59

the cellular constituents of malignant growths were 'kugelartige Zellen', vesicular cells, containing granules or a single somewhat bigger nucleus, or even entire young cells. These he looked upon as the actual 'seminium morbi' (Fig. 24).

A second type of cellular elements consisted of 'tailed bodies', which Müller regarded as connective tissue cells in an early stage of maturation. In addition, he noticed fibres and crystals. None of these elements were pathognomic, Müller admitted, so he was not able to distinguish malignant from benign processes by the mere microscopic aspect. If Müller had been careful not to commit himself, others were less reserved and came to look upon the 'tailed bodies' as typical cancer constituents.

It thus became evident, that the microscope could open new avenues for cancer research and, all over Europe, innumerable research workers started to make intensive use of it.

In 1843, the Copenhagen anatomist Adolph Hannover (1814–94), a pupil of Johannes Müller, believed that he had found a specific cancer cell, which was not a tailed body. This round or oval cell distinguished itself by a comparatively large nucleus or by several nuclei within the same cell, and by a translucent nucleolus.[171]

The existence of a characteristic cancer cell was confirmed in 1845 by Hermann Lebert (1813–78), an outstanding German pathologist of the mid-nineteenth century. He had wandered about a good deal, before he came to occupy a university chair in Zürich in 1853 and in Breslau in 1859. He spent the winters of 1842 and 1845 in Paris, in which period he published, among other things, his *Physiologie pathologique*. He could write in French as easily as in German, which enabled him to play an important part as a mediator between the German and French medical sciences. Lebert paid special attention to the cancer cell by which malignant disease would distinguish itself

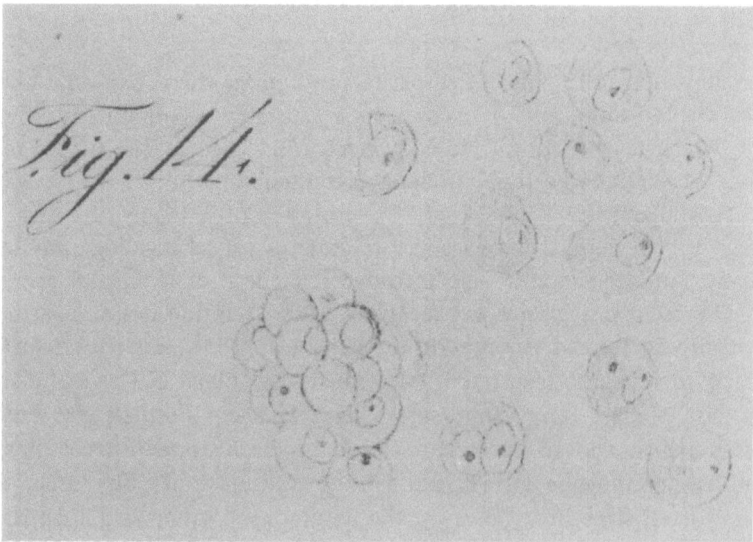

Fig. 24. Cells with germinal cells and nuclei from an extremely hard carcinoma simplex – infiltrated cancer – which had already burst open, observed by J. Müller.

from other morbid growths. He described that cell as being small and round, with an excentric, oval nucleus that occupied half or more of the lumen and contained one or more large nucleoli. This nucleus was the most characteristic part of the cancer cell.[172] In his *Traité pratique des maladies cancéreuses* at the time one of the most authoritative books on cancer and with its 892 pages probably also one of the heaviest, Lebert, in 1851, attributed the origin of cancer to imbibition of the muscle fibres and glands by the semi-fluid matrix or blastema from which the cancer cell supposedly arose. By this process the normal tissues would turn pale and disappear and be substituted by cancer mass. Cancer juice, which Lebert thought to be typical as well, would likewise proceed from cancer blastema. The latter was probably an exsudate from the blood. Lebert's supposition, that cancers arise from blastemata, was an expression of his belief in the existence of a more basic morbid condition of the blood and is strongly reminiscent of Rokitansky's doctrine of crases, which we will touch on in Chapter 7. In course of time, Lebert attached less importance to cancer juice as a distinctive feature. In his *Traité pratique*, he also mitigated somewhat his condition that a tumour might only be considered malignant if cancer cells were present. These might be absent, but no cancer occurs without a luxurious cell formation. The nuclei may be free or lying within the cells in unusual numbers.[173] Nuclei without a coating of cytoplasm and cell membrane played an important part in the histology of cancer at the time. As Haneveld pointed out, this may well have resulted from the way in which microscopic preparations were made before the introduction of the microtome; namely, by dabbing on a glass object or by plucking out with a needle. Figure 25 shows a dab-preparation of a breast cancer, recently made by Dr. Haneveld: free nuclei are indeed a feature. Unlike Johannes Müller, Lebert continued to be a clinician as well as a

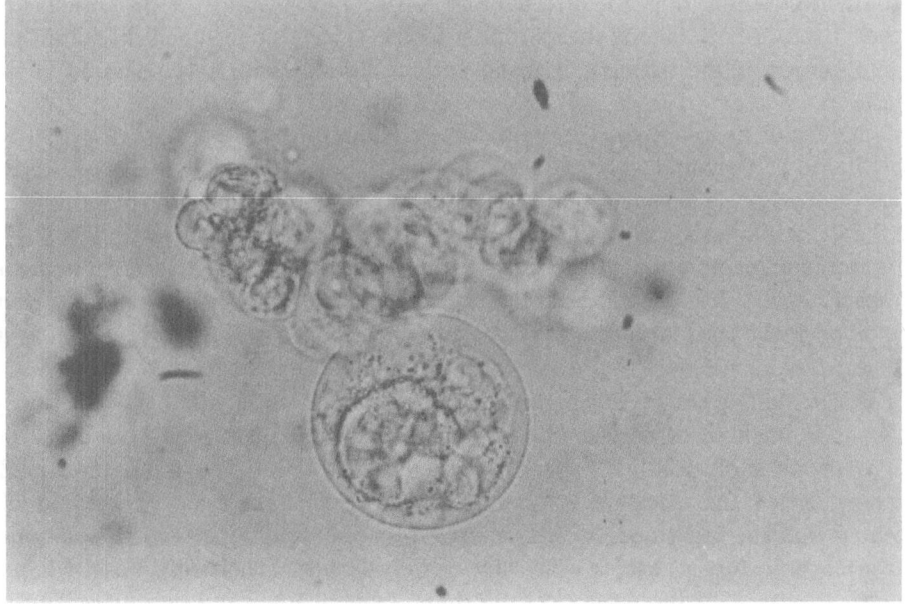

Fig. 25.   Dab-preparation of breast cancer.

pathologist. The most fertile collaboration in his Paris time was with Alfred Velpeau, successor to Boyer in La Charité. His *Nouveaux éléments de médecine opératoire* (1832) served as a guide to many generations of surgeons (Fig. 26). Velpeau was one of the greatest authorities on mammary carcinoma of the middle of the last century. In his voluminous *Traité des maladies du sein*, which appeared in 1854, he gave an excellent survey of the contemporary state of affairs, while presenting at length his own views as well.[174] In view of the importance of this book, we will give it some consideration.

Velpeau distinguished three main groups of breast cancer on the basis of external features: scirrhus, encephaloid and a fibroplastic form.[175] Many varieties existed particularly in the scirrhus: 'scirrhus ligneux, lardacé, disséminé, en plaques', etc., as well as a number of subvarieties, all of this he amply specified and described. The type of cancer which was named 'cancer encéphaloïde' or 'cancer fongeux' by Laennec, was also known as medullary cancer and was first described by William Hey (1736–1819), a surgeon in Leeds and a former student of John Hunter. He had given it the name of 'fungus haematodes'. This is, in contrast to scirrhus, a soft type of growth and particularly malignant. Hey had compared the tumour mass to brain marrow and thought that it was formed by extravasated blood and lymph, which afterwards became organized.[176] The separation of fungus from cancer in a proper sense and the great numbers of different designations given to the former tumour by all sorts of researchers, created the utmost confusion. It was also a matter of dispute whether fungus could be considered a cancer. Velpeau apparently regarded it as a species of cancer: in the 250 cases of cancer he had witnessed, there were sixty of the encephaloid type.[177]

The differential diagnosis between this tumour and scirrhus – which was also a cancer, in Velpeau's opinion – was relatively easy in the case of the breast. When scirrhus involves the skin, the affected part is drawn backward, whereas encephaloid pushes it forward.[178] Among the fibroplastic cancers Velpeau included chondroid and colloid cancers. Other species of malignant conditions very rarely occurred in the breast.

In his *Traité*, he also gave a very interesting account of the actual state of cytohistologic diagnosis.[179] Earlier in his life, Velpeau himself had for many years been trying in vain to find a 'matière cancéreuse', which he expected to occur in the blood, should the theory of diathesis – as expounded by Lebert and others – be correct.

Microscopic exploration of the pathological tissue itself had yielded more profit in recent years. It had become clear that cancerous tissue could be differentiated from any other histological structure by using the microscope. In Germany, as well as in France, many microscopists were busy trying to establish firm criteria.

The question, whether or not cancer cells contained elements that were clearly different from those in normal tissue, was an interesting one. Velpeau pointed out that German histologists like Johannes Müller, Julius Vogel (1814–80) and Rudolf Virchow denied the existence of pathognomonic cellular elements. These authors accepted that all tissues develop from certain primordial cells. This would also apply to cancer, even though cancer cells show endless varieties. Therefore, Vogel was not inclined to attach to the cancer cell the importance it was given by others. Thus it would not be possible to make the diagnosis on the appearance of a single cell. There

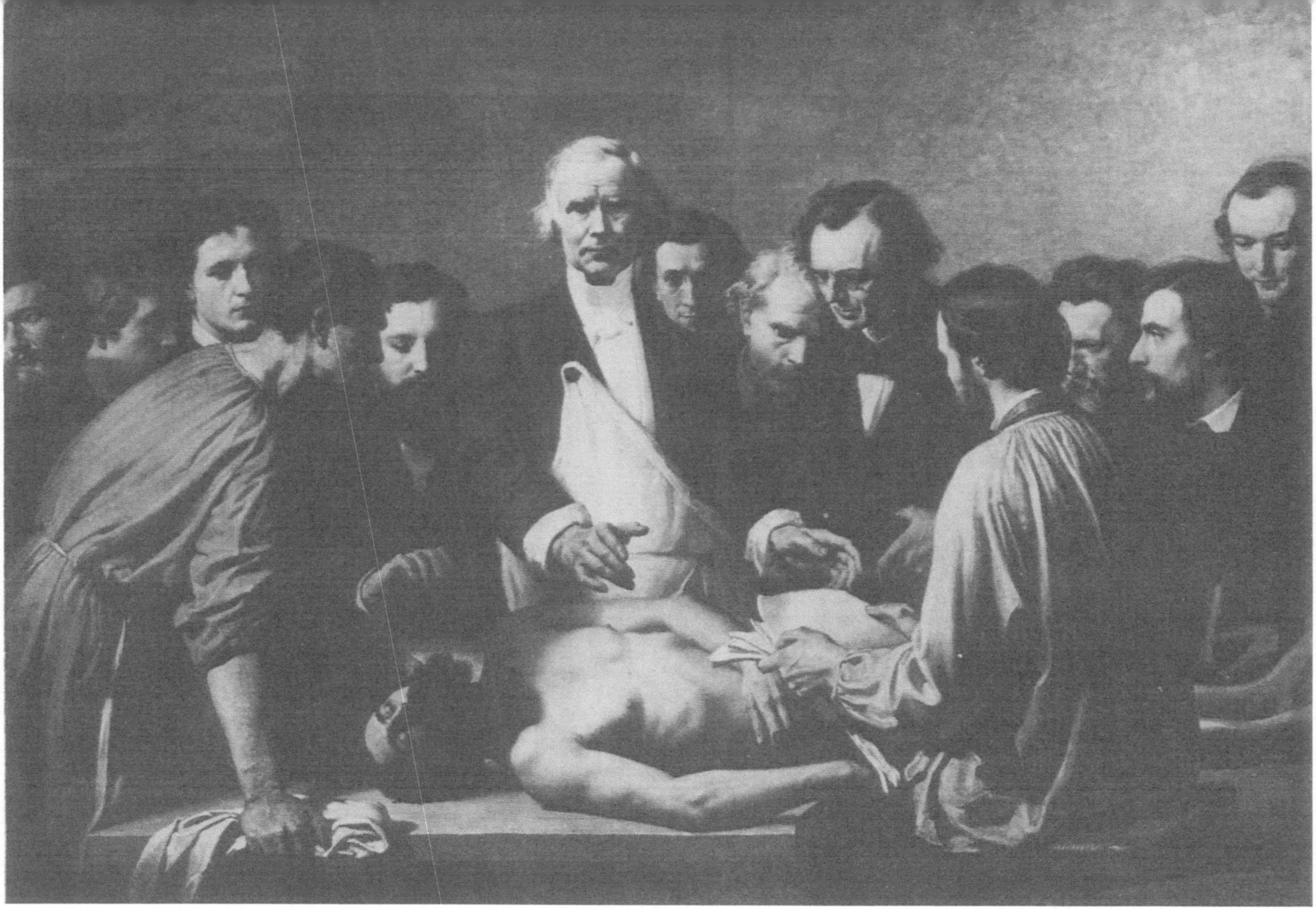

Fig. 26. A lesson by Professor Velpeau.

remained no shadow of doubt, however, when viewing a large number of such cells with all their different forms. Vogel's pronouncement seemed to represent the views of the majority of German 'micrographs'.

Virchow denied that cancer consisted of 'heterologous tissue', as Laennec had explained, and held that its elements were not basically different from those of benign tumours or of embryonic germinal tissue. Velpeau also quoted the opinion of Bennett, who had expounded that cancers of the mucous membranes, the skin and the bone were nothing but augmentations of the primitive structure. Young squamous cell epithelium, Bennett had noted, show all the features of the cancer cell. Malignant cells, however, do not have the tendency to unite into groups or to align themselves end to end, as epithelial cells are wont to do. They do not adhere and show much difference in size.

John Hughes Bennett (1812–75) was professor of clinical medicine in Edinburgh. In 1845, he had given the first clinical description of leukaemia. Velpeau took Bennett's views from his work *On cancerous and canceroid growths*, which had appeared in 1849. This book contained, among other things, a meticulous description of 56 tumours that were removed by surgery, with 190 microscopic drawings by the author. Since no copy appears to be present in any Dutch public library, the present author was not able to consult it. Velpeau was not disposed to attach any more diagnostic importance to the cancer cell than the German 'micrographs'.[180] Much of the material on which Lebert had based his conclusions had been sent to him by Velpeau. In quite a few cases, the microscopic diagnosis, made on the strength of the presence or the absence of cancer cells, had not been consistent with the clinical course. According to Velpeau, the so-called cancer cell was only a secondary product, instead of being the element 'sine qua non' of the disease. There must exist a 'more intimate' underlying principle which science would have to discover in order to be more precise about the nature of cancer. Velpeau was prepared to accept that cancer originated from an abnormal exudation and that the material differences between the species depended on the relative proportion of the material constituents of the exudative mass. Although it was obvious to Velpeau that a special predisposition for the disease existed, he did not exclude mechanical causes. Cancer is more often seen on the surface of the body — breasts, lips, testicles, eyes, orbita — than in the interior, he argued. But even internal cancers occur especially at sites exposed to chemical or mechanical irritation: mouth, pharynx, oesophagus, both orifices of the stomach, anus, rectum, neck of the urinary bladder, cervix uteri. Contrary to public opinion, he did not consider sorrow and fear to be of carcinogenic impact.

The well-established fact that cachexia only occurs some time after the appearance of a primary tumour was sufficient proof that cancer had a local origin. In Velpeau's view, carcinoma comes into being first because of a small infiltration of blood, albumen, plastic material. Such an infiltration may be the effect of either external or internal — travail moleculaire — influences. This mass turns into a foreign body in which new life can establish itself, with the consequence that the tumour acquires its own existence.[181] It is somewhat surprising to see, all of a sudden, a vitalistic element appear in Velpeau's pathology, and that, at a time when scientific materialism had already gained a firm foot in medicine.

The French Académie de Médecine refused to accept the existence of a specific cancer cell at its 1854 meeting, which was entirely devoted to the problem of cancer. Although the leading spirits of France exchanged their views — sometimes in heated debate — for thirteen sessions in succession, they failed to define the microscopic features of malignancy.[182]

CHAPTER 7

Scientific developments in the second half
of the nineteenth century

About the middle of the last century microscopical research in France was directed in particular at pathologic cytology, whilst in Germany, where Johannes Müller's school was predominant, more attention was being paid to the structure of the diseased tissues. At the same time, German research workers displayed great interest in the genesis of cancer: where do the first cancer cells come from? They first focussed attention on blastema, the matrix of all cells as was generally accepted in the 1840's and still adhered to by many even in the fifties.

In 1845, Julius Vogel, professor of pathology in Halle, whom we discussed previously when he was cited by Velpeau, described blastema as a solid, amorphous substance which resembled coagulated fibrin and was, in fact, most probably fibrin.[183] Karl Rokitansky (1804—78) in Vienna, to whom, although we are no longer aware of it, we owe a substantial part of our present-day pathologico-anatomic knowledge, was at first also a partisan of the blastema theory: blastema was regarded as a derivate of blood serum and was assumed to ooze continuously from the blood vessels. Carcinoma would, in Rokitansky's opinion, be pre-existent in impaired blood as a particular 'crasis', which could engender a particular blastema.

However much Rokitansky was used to thinking in solidistic and morphological categories, in the last analysis he ascribed disease to the morbid conditions of the blood, of albumin in particular. Diseased albumin was seen as the material cause of the most dangerous local growth that can be met with within the body.[184] It is certainly curious to find, once again, a humoral-pathologic tendency in the theories of one of the most outstanding pathologists of the last century, in a time when ancient humoral pathology had definitely had its day and was being replaced by solidistic views. But Rokitansky was certainly not the only author expressing such views half way the nineteenth century. We have already noted the carcinogenic significance which Lebert attached to blastema as an exsudate from the blood and Sir James Paget (1814—99), surgeon to St. Bartholomew's Hospital in London and an outstanding pathologist, remembered for his disease of the nipple, seems to have more or less shared Rokitansky's hypothesis as late as 1863, although he did not acknowledge it. In his well-known *Lectures on surgical pathology*, in which he gave, amongst many other things, excellent expositions on scirrhous, medullary cancer and colloid cancer of the breast, he held that cancers are '...local manifestations of certain specific morbid states of the blood; and that in them are incorporated peculiar

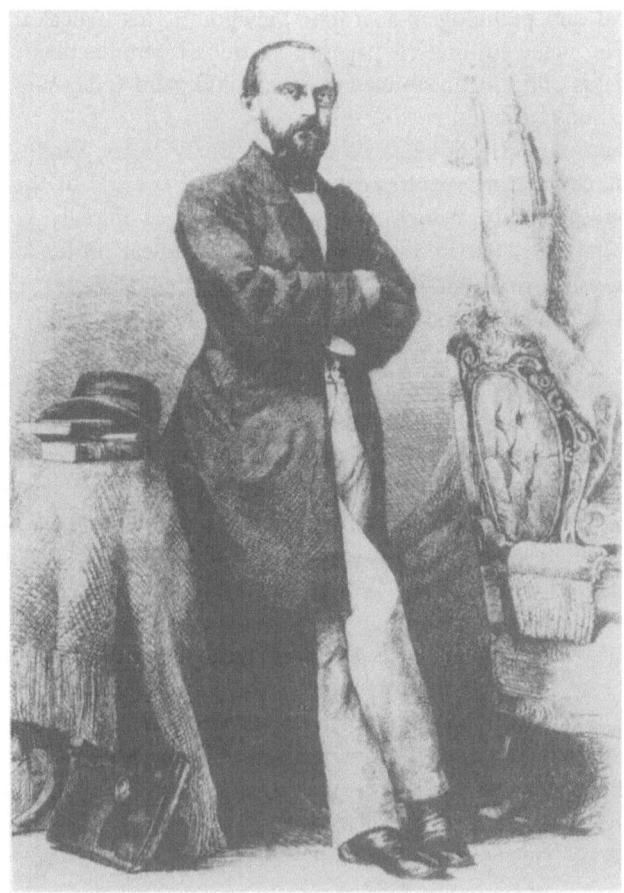

Fig. 27. Rudolf Virchow in 1862.

morbid materials which accumulate in the blood, and which their growth may tend to increase'.[185] This statement is all the more surprising since Rokitansky's doctrine of crases had been fiercely attacked years before by the young Rudolf Virchow (1821–1902) in one of his first published articles (Fig. 27).

In his master work, *Die Cellularpathologie* (1858), the great champion of solidistic pathology had advanced that the cell is the bearer of life, and therefore also of disease. Disease is life under altered conditions, a reaction of the cell to abnormal stimuli.[186] As to the genesis of cells, Virchow agreed with Robert Remak (1815–65), professor of anatomy in Berlin, who in 1852 was the first to point out that the growth of tissues was accomplished by the division of pre-existing cells.[187] The biological principle of 'omnis cellula e cellula', as it was formulated at the time, became of paramount importance for the further development of pathology.

For our purpose, however, another of Virchow's works is of more importance – his *Die krankhaften Geschwülste*, which appeared in three volumes between 1863 and

1867. The way in which Virchow, in this book, approached the cancer problem from historical, clinical and pathologico-anatomic viewpoints, his logical train of thought and his clear style, make turning the pages of his book a genuine pleasure, even today. Quite a view of his pungent pronouncements are still valid today and this applies to Virchow's entire body of work.

As to the microscopical activities of the past thirty years, Virchow recalled that nothing short of designating specific cancer cells was expected of the microscopists. Certain ideas on specificity, which research workers had initially been careful not to suggest, had taken shape in the minds of the medical profession. Thus it was fashionable, for some time, to look upon Müller's 'tailed bodies' as characteristic cancer elements. Whenever something is established consensu omnium in science, it is very hard to remove it again. Apparently, since the zoologists' crawfish have tails, many were inclined to mark the pathologists' cancers with similar extensions.[188]

The foundations for any consideration of the problem had already been laid by Bichat, who, Virchow wrote, had divided tumours into two basic categories: those having analogy with familiar parts of the body and those possessing a divergent structure. This division had not been made by Bichat, however, but by Laennec. Virchow, too, distinguished a homologous group of tumours, characterized by proliferation of cells that were already present, from a heterologous group in which the growth is made up of tissue abnormal to the part. The first group is usually benign, the second one, as a rule, malignant. Although tumours belonging to the latter class behave like parasites, they still form part of the body and do not arise from any arbitrary juice. The laws of the body apply just as well to the tumour.[189]

Curiously, Virchow attributed the origin of all malignant growths to heterologous changes of connective tissue[190] (Fig. 28). In this respect, he agreed with the views expressed by Bichat in 1901 and by Grashuys as early as 1741! He did not go into the actual cause of cancer in any length, imputing it rather vaguely to 'chronic irritation'.[191]

A number of years before, Virchow had postulated a connective tissue origin with regard to cancroid. In 1854, he had already been attacked on that point by Robert Remak, a former pupil of Johannes Müller and subsequently the originator of the important germ-layer theory. Remak held the belief that cancroid developed exclusively from epidermic cells.[192] His views were confirmed in 1865 by thorough microscopical investigations carried out by Carl Thiersch (1822–95), professor of surgery in Erlangen.[193] In 1872, Wilhelm von Waldeyer-Hartz (1865–1921), professor of pathological anatomy in Breslau, established the epithelial origin of *all* types of cancer.[194] It should be noted that, in the meantime, histological research had been considerably facilitated by the introduction of staining methods. The microtome was not yet available, however, and these investigators still cut their sections by hand. Thiersch and Waldeyer had based their theoretical considerations, to a great extent, on Remak's germ-layer doctrine, from which they concluded that epithelial cells can develop only from epithelium.

In the next few years, rapid developments took place in the microscopical diagnosis of cancer. Instead of homology and heterology, typical or atypical features, maturity or immaturity and all their many states of transition became the standards on which

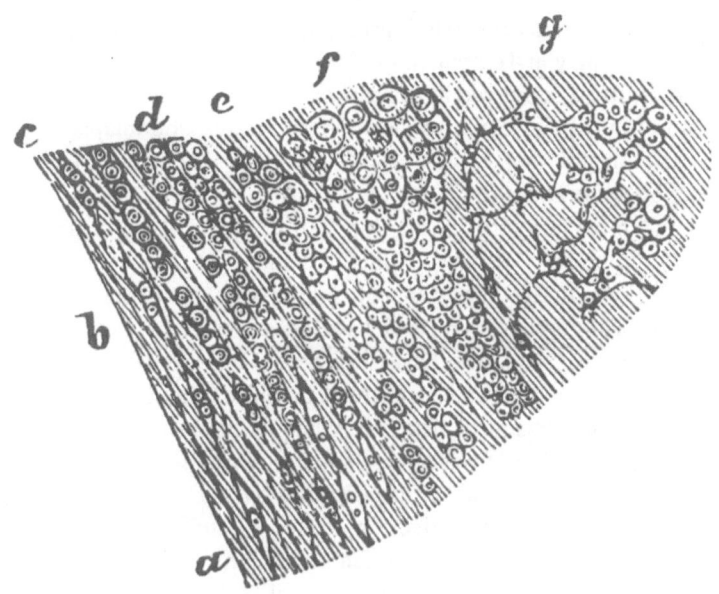

Fig. 28. Development of cancer from connective tissue in carcinoma mammae, according to Virchow.

a Connective tissue corpuscles   e Enlargement of the young cells and nests
b Cell fission   f Further enlargement of cells and nests
c Mitosis   g The same development in cross section
d Filing in of the cells

judgement was based. Carcinoma was coming to be understood as a neoplasm made up of epithelium and sarcoma as a tumour arising from connective tissue.[195] Towards the end of the century, professor Hermann Tillmans (1844–1927) in Leipzig gave the following definition of cancer: 'Cancer is a new growth developing from finished epithelial epidermic and glandular cells, which disturbs the normal tissue type of the primarily diseased part of the body. It is characterized by unlimited peripheral growth, by epithelial metastases particularly along the lymph vessels, more rarely along the blood vessels, and ends mortally in the great majority of cases under the symptoms of a general intoxication'.[196] Ninety years later, we have but little to add.

It was not only the more minute structures of tumours, which kept research workers intensively busy in the second half of the century; the question of the aetiology of cancer also received much attention. The hypotheses of Julius Cohnheim and of Hugo Ribbert became well-known. Cohnheim (1839–84), one of the great teachers of pathology in the nineteenth century, had been a pupil of Virchow, before he became professor of pathological anatomy in Kiel, Breslau and Leipzig successively. He traced the fundamental cause of cancer to an error in the embryonic development. At a very early stage, groups of cells would separate from their normal coherence and lie dormant for an indefinite time. Later in life, such 'versprengte Keime' could start festering. According to Ribbert (1855–1920) in Bonn, the essential feature was not the embryonic character of the cells, but the separation in adult life of basically normal cells from their natural relationship, that would engender their independant growth.[197] David Paul von Hansemann (1858—1920) in Berlin held the opinion that the asymmetric mitosis, observed in the cancer cell, would cause the loss of its specific properties and entail the creation of an undifferentiated and anaplastic element with an increased growth potency. Proliferation took place when such anaplastic cells had been activated by some stimulus.[198]

The triumphs of bacteriology in isolating, within a short lapse of time, the causative germs of many infectious diseases, stimulated many to look diligently for a living cancer agent.[199] Such an agent was expected to belong not to the bacteria, but rather to the protozoa. This feeling may well have been aroused by the discovery of the malarial plasmodium by Alphonse Laveran (1845—1922) in 1880. The research along this line produced an extensive literature. The infectious theory in the genesis of cancer lost much of its attraction, however, when in 1903 the Copenhagen pathologist Carl Oluf Jensen (1864—1934) was able to show that mouse cancer can be transmitted by tissue transplantation through 22 generations. That his outcome was really based on transplantation, and not on infection, followed sufficiently from the fact that inoculation with smashed cells always turned out negative.[200]

The way in which metastasis takes place was also the object of much research and much difference of opinion. In the eighteenth century there was a suspicion that the disease was spread throughout the body by a poisonous or tainted humour, but Johannes Müller quite rightly concluded, from his solidistic conceptions, that cells with a tendency to reproduction might enter into the circulation and give rise to tumour growth elsewhere in the body. He wondered whether cancerous masses in the veins, as observed by Cooper, Cruveilhier and others, had anything to do with the dissemination of cancer.

Others did not attribute the transfer to cancer cells themselves, but to the blastema from which such elements proceed. 'A rudimental liquid, an unformed cancerous blastema, mingled with the blood, may be effectual as any germs', wrote Sir James Paget.[201]

It is worthy of note that even Virchow in his *Die krankhafte Geschwülste* still adhered, to some extent, to a humoral explanation. He presumed that dissemination was favoured by a relative abundance of parenchymatous juices in the pathologic growth. The drier a neoplasm, the smaller the chance of proximal or distant infection. Virchow believed that transfer of the juices takes place by way of the lymphatics. The tumour may also affect the walls of veins. These become cancerous and after some time the process penetrates into the lumen of the vessel as a cancer plug. It is only in the veins that material cancer particles can move elsewhere. Absorption of cancer cells in the lymphatics is not absolutely impossible, but can only occur when the lymph nodes themselves have become entirely cancerous. A peripheral lymph vessel can never simply carry cells from the tumour to the blood. The familiar observation that, in the case of breast cancer, the lungs are far less frequently involved than the liver, argues against the supposition that the disease is transferred by material particles. Apparently, cancer juices have the ability to induce the same tumours elsewhere as those from which they proceed. Thiersch and Waldeyer also contested this one notion propounded by Virchow, arguing that cancer cells transfer the disease either by a process of embolisation or by continuous growth.

70

Stephen Paget in London, not to be confused with Sir James Paget, was of the opinion that the dissemination of cancer cells occurred at random, but that the specific distribution of metastases to the organs was by no means arbitrary. In 1889, he wrote that, in 735 cases of mammary carcinoma, he had found 241 instances of metastases in the liver and only 17 in the spleen, which has a rich blood supply all the same. Some organs apparently constitute a favourable matrix for the emboli, whereas, in others, the deposited cells are destroyed.[202]

Heredity continued to attract the interest of pathologists and clinicians. It goes without saying that those who attached significance to 'predisposition' in the genesis of cancer, were more inclined than others to accept the existence of heredity. Conversely, James Paget defended his views on the constitutional condition for cancer by, amongst other things, giving a striking instance of a cancer family. 'A lady died with cancer of the stomach, one of her daughters died with cancer of the stomach, another died with cancer of the breast, and of her grandchildren, two died of cancer of the breast, two of cancer of the uterus, one of cancer of the bladder, one of cancer of the axillary glands, one of cancer of the stomach, one of cancer of the rectum! Now, it seems to me inconceivable that we can here speak of the transmission of anything local'.[203]

Paul Broca (1824–1880), a surgical pathologist in Paris, who, however, earned a world reputation as an anthropologist, published in 1852, together with his father-in-law, the physician Georges-Antoine Lugol (1786–1851), the pedigree of a family which had itself produced three famous doctors. Within four generations, 16 of its 27 members had died from cancer, of the breast (11), of the liver (3), of the stomach (1) and of the uterus (1), respectively. This sad genealogy is reprinted in Wolff.[204] Yet another 'cancer family' was presented by Charles Hewitt Moore, to whom we will turn our attention in Chapter 9.

CHAPTER 8

Mammary carcinoma in the light
of new developments

The preceding chapter discussed the developments in general cancerology, especially in the latter half of the last century, so we will now examine the consequences which these advancements had for the diagnosis and nosology of breast cancer.

For this purpose we might well consult a book by Billroth, *Die Krankheiten der Brustdrüse*, first issued in 1880.[205] Theodor Billroth (1824–67) was professor of surgery, first in Zürich (1860–67) and subsequently in Vienna. He belonged to that heroic generation of surgeons who, only a few decades after the introduction of antisepsis in 1864, raised surgery from a traditional craft to a scientific discipline. Billroth, one of the founders of abdominal surgery, was also an outstanding pathologist.

According to Billroth, the morphological diagnosis of cancer had lately gained so much in reliability, that it offered at least as much certainty as the clinical signs elaborated through the ages. The clinical and anatomical features coincided fairly accurately by now. Many authors had recently tried to develop a classification. In this, some had gone much further than others and, since the different kinds of tumour sometimes had different names in different countries, confusion threatened to arise where a clear view was, in fact, badly needed.

Billroth tried to put things in order by accepting only four kinds of breast cancer. For survey purposes, he drew up a vocabulary in which he listed both his own nomenclature and the names in common use that had been given to the same type of tumour by others. As representatives of those whose set of terms had become widely known, he chose his predecessor at the Viennese chair Franz Schuh (1804–65), John Birkett (1815–1904), surgeon to Guy's Hospital in London, Samuel David Gross (1805–84), professor of surgery at Louisville and Jefferson Medical College in the United States, and Velpeau in Paris, whom we discussed previously. Billroth's table is valuable even today for the student of historical oncology.[206]

I. *Die theils weicheren, theils härteren Carcinomknoten*: histologisch meist als acinöses Carcinom auftretend (Billroth).
   Identical with: Markschwamm (medullary fungus).
   Schuh: Faserkrebs mit grossen Knoten.
   Birkett: Carcinoma medullare. Encysted carcinoma. Lobular carcinoma, attached to or involving only one lobe. Tuberous form of cancer.

72

Gross: Encephaloid. Tuberous form of cancer.

Velpeau: Encéphaloïde. Squirrhe proprement dit ou globuleux.

II. *Die carcinomatöse Infiltration:* histologisch meist als tubulöses Carcinom auftretend. Carcinoma simplex (Billroth). Usually spreading at an early stage to the skin, partly as an infiltration, partly as multiple nodules.

Schuh: Faserkrebs mit kleinen Knoten. Linsenförmiger Krebs.

Birkett: Intra-glandular carcinoma. Infiltrating form of cancer.

Gross: Infiltrating form of cancer.

Velpeau: all his types of 'squirrhe': squirrhe ligneux (having the density and inextensibility of wood), s. rayonné ou rameux, s. tégumentaire ou en cuirasse, s. en masse, en nappe, s. disséminé ou pustuleux, s. lardacé. Kéloïdes (Fig. 29).

III. *Der atrophirende, vernarbende Brustkrebs:* Scirrhus (Billroth).

Gross: Atrophic scirrhus.

Velpeau: Squirrhe rétractile ou atrophique.

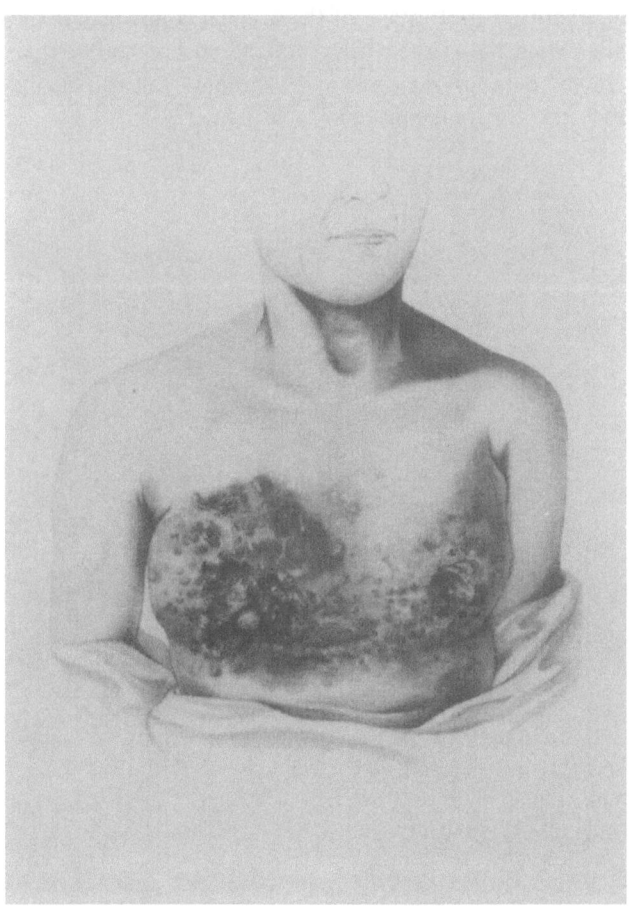

Fig. 29.   One of Billroth's patients.

IV. *Gallertkrebs*:
    Gross: Glatiniform carcinoma.
    Velpeau: Squirrhe gélatineux, alvéolaire. Cancer colloide.

By means of fine woodcuts, Billroth gave a detailed description of the gross and micro-scopic features of each one of his four species. Typical of mammary cancer is the acinar appearance which, although it may also be observed in tumours elsewhere in the body, is particularly characteristic for neoplasms of the breast. The acini and tubuli are filled with large, round and irregular cells — cancer cells — which contain large nuclei, each with a strikingly shining nucleolus. The intermediate connective tissue is infiltrated by much smaller cells (Fig. 30). It was not quite clear to Billroth what the correlation between the two groups of cells might be.

The Viennese professor showed himself a supporter of the doctrine of the epithelial origin of carcinoma and he carefully explained the arguments both in favour of and against it. As to the way in which the cancer stroma arises, one of the great issues at the time, Billroth took the view that its development was not a matter of neoplasia, but that it came about by infiltration of the original connective tissue of the gland by proliferating cells. Thus the stroma was, in fact, nothing other than disrupted con-nective tissue. In his descriptions of cancer histology, Billroth also paid attention to the dynamic processes which take place in such tissue.[207]

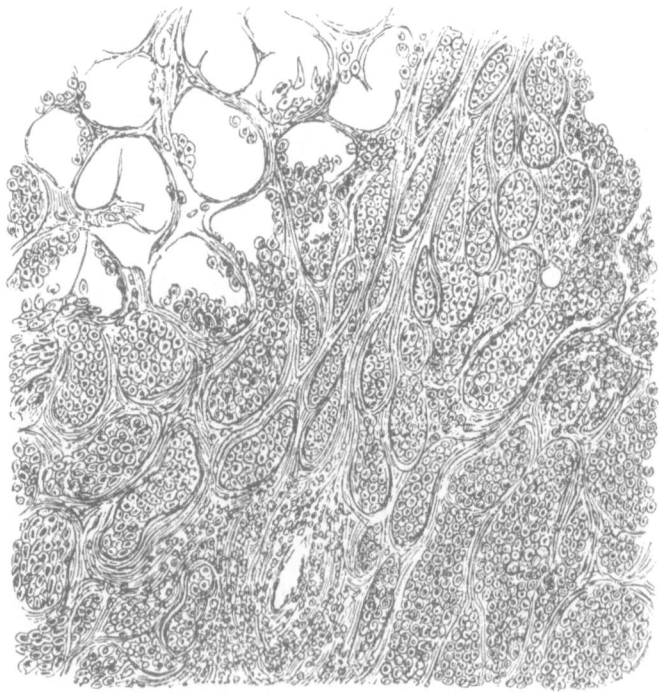

Fig. 30.   Typical aspect of mammary cancer.

With regard to the metastases of mammary cancer, Billroth confessed that he had never been able to identify in them the features of the original lesion. Yet he thought it highly probable that metastasis would take place by the spread of corpuscular elements by means of the lymphatics. In all cases of disseminated breast cancer he had been able to observe that the regional lymph nodes were always involved. Lymphatics in the pleura and on the diaphragm repeatedly appeared to be filled with carcinoma cells. He also believed in the possibility of metastatic spread through the veins, although he had as yet failed to find anatomical evidence. The microcellular elements in the intermediate connective tissue were assigned the same potencies of spreading as the proper carcinoma cells. It was generally accepted at the time that carcinoma was, as its inception, purely a local disease with a solitary origin which infected the body from the primary site. Secondary growths of breast cancer occurred particularly in the liver, followed, in order of diminishing frequency, by the pleurae and the lungs, the bones and the brains. Billroth herewith confirmed the experience reported by Birkett in 1850, who had treated 37 cases at Guy's Hospital in London. In contrast to Birkett, however, Billroth had never observed metastatic foci in the ovaries or the uterus. Of much interest are also Billroth's descriptions of the clinical course of mammary carcinoma.[208] In this he relied to a considerable degree on statistical data.

As long as medicine used qualitative ways of thinking, weight and measures and numbers were of relatively little importance as scientific categories. Towards the end of the eighteenth century there had been a change in this. We have already noted the work of Monro and Hill, who by means of series of numbers tried to evaluate the value of operative treatment. The value of the numerical method became fully appreciated when in 1806, E. Duvillard in Paris, applying a primitive statistical analysis, showed the favourable effect of smallpox vaccination on the general mortality rate.[209] In addition, his fellow-townsman, Pierre-Charles-Alexandre Louis (1787–1872), by adopting a similar approach, exposed the futility of therapeutic bloodletting in 1835.[210] Before long, statistics began to play an important part in the study of cancer. An outstanding medical statistician at the time was Domenico Antonio Rigoni-Stern (1810–18?), provincial surgeon of Verona in Italy. The paper that he presented at the Subsession on Surgery of the Fourth Congress of Italian Scientists in 1842, was rescued from oblivion by Scotto and Bailar in 1969.[211] Rigoni-Stern's methods, which he used in collecting, analysing and presenting statistical data, were not very dissimilar to those in use today. His data were collected from death registries from the city and suburbs of Verona for the 80-year period from 1760 to 1839 inclusive, and covered an overall number of 150,673 deaths. From his studies he concluded, according to Scotto and Bailar, among other things, that:
— the incidence of cancer generally increases with age;
— the increase is mainly due to a rapid increase in uterine cancers;
— the frequency of breast cancer is inversely related to the incidence of uterine cancer for different age groups;
— unmarried persons generally have a greater chance of contracting cancer, especially breast cancer in women;
— married women contract uterine cancer more often than unmarried women;
— cancer of different anatomical sites probably has different aetiologies.

Billroth had his huge material of cancer cases statistically analysed by his assistant Alexander von Winiwarter (1848–1917), who had become professor of surgery in Liege, Belgium, in 1878.[212] From this analysis it appeared that the first of Billroth's four groups, medullary carcinoma, has the most rapid course and is more apt to occur in younger women of about 35 to 40 years of age. Carcinoma simplex is the most frequent, but takes a very varying clinical course. Fast advancing neoplasms occur particularly in young individuals between 30 and 40 in good general condition. They first appear as an infiltrative induration which extends rapidly and, before long, occupies the greater part of the breast. After six to eight months, there is an enlargement of the axillary nodes, followed by the appearance of supraclavicular deposits. Neuralgic pains arise in the ipsilateral arm, in which, because of compression of the axillary vein, indurated oedema develops.[213] Ulceration only takes place after 1 to 1½ years. The state of nutrition remains good for a long while. Metastases develop in the pleura at the diseased side, in the liver, in the long bones and, not infrequently, in the vertebrae. The patient is now in great agony from which death will relieve her after two or three years at most.

More slowly progressing instances of carcinoma simplex are attended by early involvement of the overlying skin. Skin phenomena predominate the subsequent development in such cases. Separate nodules arise – frequently preceded by radiating hyperaemia – and progress to the point of ulceration. The skin induration spreads in all directions until finally a large area of the thorax is covered with thickened and hardened skin with nodules and ulcers (Fig. 29), a desperate condition which was aptly described as 'cancer en cuirasse' by Velpeau twelve years before, in his well-known book. Repeated haemorrhages occur and there is loss of weight, but deposits in internal organs are late and restricted. The total duration may vary from three to six or eight years, or even longer.

A comparable slow course is taken by colloid cancer. The most benign is, however, the atrophied, scarred scirrhous carcinoma. The ulceration that may accompany it sometimes heals after the shedding of necrotic tissue, at least for some time. The superficial axillary nodes are slightly enlarged, but very firm. Billroth did not know how long such conditions could exist before they killed the patient, but he knew of old women who had carried breast indurations for more than twenty years before they died from other causes. He did not express an opinion on the matter of distant metastasis in this group of patients. They will rarely have been subjected to post-mortem examinations since Billroth did not operate upon them and therefore did not admit them to hospital.

Billroth felt able to relate the clinical behaviour of a tumour to its histologic type, yet he did not make any effort to adopt a system of clinical staging. He did not have much to say on the aetiology of mammary cancer either. He pointed out that the breasts, just like the internal sexual organs, rapidly undergo functional developments during puberty and pregnancy, and wondered if their very adaptibility might be the reason that they are more prone to the development of autonomous growths than organs that function steadily throughout life. Unfortunately, it was not then possible to produce genuine experimental tumours. The specific nature of the particular stimuli which gave occasion to neoplasia or, conversely, the state in which the tissue has to be in order for it to produce morbid growths under the influence of normal, familiar stimuli, was not known.[214]

In accordance with the long-standing belief in an individual predispostion for chronic inflammatory diseases like scrophulosis and tuberculosis, Billroth accepted the existence of a particular innate cancer diathesis. Both diatheses do not fully exclude one another, but it is quite rare to find cancer and tuberculosis combined in one individual.[215] The belief that cancer and tuberculosis are mutually preclusive was first advanced by Caspar-Laurent Bayle (1774–1816) and Jean-Bruno Cayol (1787–1856), in their extensive chapter on cancer in the *Dictionnaire des Sciences Médicales* in 1812.[160] In 1846 Rokitansky in Vienna expressed a similar view.[216] When studying the death-rates of cancer in England and Wales, the English physician John Francis Churchill called attention to the fact that in the three decades preceeding 1885, an increase of 74 per cent in the mortality caused by cancer was accompanied by a corresponding decrease of 60 per cent in the mortality from phtisis.[217]

In Churchill's opinion, tuberculosis was caused by a deficiency of 'oxydizable phosphorus', the chief initiator of cell growth. Some twenty years before, he had, accordingly, started to treat consumption with hypophosphites and his remarkable successes had induced many physicians to imitate his example. Indeed, phosphorus compounds had become quite fashionable in therapeutics and were, at the time, amongst the ingredients of many invigorating and strengthening medicines, foods, beverages and tonics.

This had resulted in a rapid decrease of tuberculosis, but since cancer depended upon the contrary condition — an excess of the 'phosphide element' — it had increased the number of cancer victims at the same time.

In his long-winded paper, Dr. Churchill offered no explanation of the fact that female cancer mortality had increased in a larger proportion than male mortality (Fig. 31). Churchill was by no means the only, or even the first physician to draw attention to an increase in cancer. In 1823, Anton Friedrich Fischer (1778–1839) in Breslau remarked, in the opening sentence of a paper on glandular diseases of the

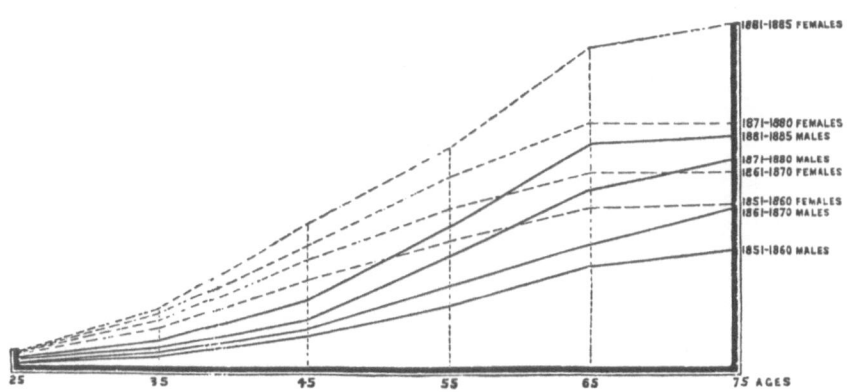

Fig. 31. Increase of cancer deaths in England and Wales for each of the sexes between 1851 and 1885, described by J.F. Churchill.

female bosom, that beginning and advanced indurations in the breasts of the fair sex were occurring more frequently than ever.[218] An interesting survey of the return of cancer deaths in Würzburg between 1852 and 1855, very carefully made by Virchow in person, gave no answer to the question of any increase in the mortality of malignant diseases, since it only related to three years. It did show, however, that, at the time, breast cancer was certainly not the most conspicuous form of human cancer:[219]

Stomach	34.9%
Uterus, vagina, etc.	18.5%
Large and small intestines	8.1%
Liver, etc.	7.5%
Face, lips	4.9%
Mammary glands	4.3%

The Belgian Bernard Eduard vanden Corput (1821–1908), writing in 1883, mentioned in passing the increasing cancer mortality in London and Vienna in an article in which he discussed the nature of cancer diathesis. By diathesis he understood a special pathogenic predisposition; it is interesting to note that he imputed that condition to an incorrect diet.[220]

Neither Churchill, nor vanden Corput furnished a statement as to the composition of their cancer populations. Cancer mortality in Amsterdam between 1862 and 1902 was discussed with much detail in an interesting report published by the statistical bureau of that town in 1908.[221] It appears that the mortality caused by cancer showed a regular increase since 1862. The report expresses no opinion as to whether the statistic augmentation represents a real increase or is due to an improvement in diagnosis. In any case, cancer mortality had shown no decrease, as had been the case in many other causes of death, like tuberculosis. As regards cancer of the breast and of the uterus, the increase between 1862 and 1902 had been slight, from 2.9 to 3.2 per 10,000 inhabitants. Cancer in women of the alimentary tract had increased in the same period from 2.6 to 5.8 per 10,000.

CHAPTER 9

Surgical treatment in the second half
of the nineteenth century

Important factors that contributed to surgery taking the premier place in the treatment of breast cancer in the latter half of the nineteenth century were the introduction of surgical anaesthesia in 1846, the triumph of the solidistic concept with regard to carcinogenesis, the adoption of antiseptic principles in 1864 (Fig. 32) and the steadily increasing refinement of surgical technique.

Few inventions have spread over the globe as swiftly as inhalation anaesthesia. Within a year after the dentist William Thomas Green Morton (1819–68) in Boston had made the first important American contribution to medicine by his discovery of the anaesthetic effects of sulphuric ether, the procedure was applied all over the Western world. In Europe it was used in countries as far removed from one another as Russia and Scotland. In the latter country, James Syme in Glasgow, whom we know already as the surgeon of Ailie Noble, was one of its early champions. Johann Friedrich Dieffenbach (1792–1847), professor in Berlin and one of the founders of plastic surgery, referred to etherisation, in his book *Operative Chirurgie*,[222] as 'a veritable treasure', when explaining the extirpation of the mammary gland and the concomitant axillary nodes. The introduction of anaesthesia, as such, did not markedly increase the frequency of mastectomy. The danger of wound infection was of course not allayed by it, the public at large had not yet forgotten the fear of pain and many medical men were not convinced of the benefit of that operation. The pessimism of the medical world was partly due to the unfavourable operative results and partly prompted by the belief in the existence of a particular diathesis. One of the pre-eminent mid-century oncologists who might be cited in this connection was Hermann Lebert, the pathologist whom we discussed in Chapter 7. It is true that he no longer upheld the classical conception of diathesis, but he assumed the existence of a cancer blastema, which had its origin in the blood. The 1854 congress of the Académie de Médecine, which was referred to in chapter 6, not only occupied itself with the minute structure of cancer, but also discussed the question of whether, as a matter of principle, cancer should be treated at all.[223] Joseph-François Malgaigne (1806–65), well known for his work on fractures, was amongst those who deemed cancer to be a quite incurable disease, whereas Velpeau, starting from the conception that cancer has a local inception, was in favour of an operative approach. It was important though, to operate as early as possible. This view was shared by the majority of the visitors to the congress. The year before in his *Maladies du sein*, Velpeau had

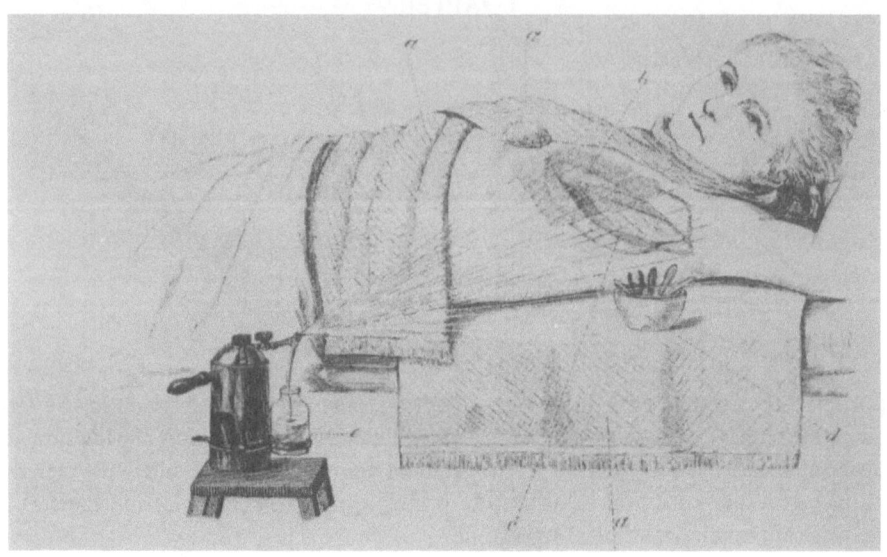

Fig. 32. Antiseptic mastectomy.

claimed to have seen more than one thousand breast tumours, benign as well as malignant in his practice of forty years standing. Only a small minority had been available for follow-up until the end: 'Once the tumour has been actually excised and the wound has healed, the surgeon and the patient easily lose sight of one another'. Yet he felt he had cured a good many cases.[224]

Statistical returns that became available about the middle of the century, however, did not appear to support Velpeau's optimism. In 1844, Jean-Jacques-Joseph Leroy d'Etiolles (1798–1860) organised an inquiry, by means of a circular, to which he received 174 answers. From these data it followed that 18 out of 1192 patients, who had not been subjected to operation, had lived for more than 30 years whilst the remainder survived from 2 to 25 years. Out of 804 that were treated by surgery, only 4 were still alive after 30 years, 15 patients had survived their operation for more than 20 years, 88 for 6 to 20 years. The conclusion was that operative treatment was more harmful than beneficial.[225]

In 1852, James Paget had come to a similar conclusion as far as scirrhus was concerned. Women who had been operated upon because of scirrhous carcinoma had, on average, died thirteen months earlier than those who had not been subjected to surgical intervention. His statistical returns concerned 60 patients, excluding those who had died as an immediate result of the operation. Sufferers from medullary cancers – not of the breast alone – on the other hand, lived for 34 months on average after operation, whereas those who had not been operated upon rarely lived for longer than one year after the outbreak of the disease. It became more and more apparent than the results of surgery bore a relationship to the histologic type of tumour.[226]

In the same year in which Joseph Lister first reported on antiseptic wound treatment, 1867, Charles Hewitt Moore (1821–70), surgeon to the Middlesex and to St. Luke's hospitals in London, formulated the general principles on which surgical treatment of mammary carcinoma should rest.[227] A standardised operation did not, as yet, exist. Some surgeons only removed the lump; others cut out the segment of the breast in which the tumour was situated or began with excision of the central mass and removed successive portions of doubtful soundness afterwards; yet others amputated the entire breast, sometimes, however, preserving a substantial skinflap which might even include the nipple. These were the operations that had been carried out by a number of surgeons on 14 patients who presented themselves in the Middlesex Hospital because of recurrences near the wounds or the scars. Amongst these patients was a woman from a family of six sisters, five of whom and their mother suffered from cancer of the left breast. From a close analysis of these cases, Moore concluded that recurrences are always due to incomplete operations and arise from local conditions. The one important point, therefore, was to carry out an adequate removal. This implies that:

It is not sufficient to remove the tumour, or any portion of the breast in which it is situated; mammary cancer requires the careful extirpation of the whole organ.

Where any texture adjoining the breast is involved in or even approached by the disease, that texture should be removed with the breast. This observation relates especially to skin, to lymphatics, to fat, and to pectoral muscle.

In the performance of that operation it is desirable to avoid, not only cutting into the tumour, but even exposing it.

Diseased axillary glands should be taken away by the same dissection as the breast itself, without dividing the intervening lymphatics.

Moore was not the first, however, to lay down the above-mentioned desideratum. As early as 1844, Joseph Pancoast (1805–82), professor of anatomy and surgery at Jefferson Medical College in Philadelphia, had recommended 'that the breast and glands should all be removed in one piece'.[228] In the next few years, mastectomy became gradually standardised in accordance with Moore's general recommendations, although this development was probably not directly inspired by him, since his paper was not very often quoted.

New developments started in Germany, where the method proposed in 1875 by the Halle professor Richard von Volkmann (1830–89) was soon followed by many. Volkmann always removed the entire breast, no matter how small the primary tumour might be. He also routinely removed the pectoral fascia, since microscopic inspection had shown that delicate carcinous extensions might reach that structure and spread over it, even if the tumour was still freely movable over the thoracic wall. Should the process have already penetrated into the muscle, a thick layer of it should be sliced off and removed as well. There were surgeons, however, who bluntly separated the breast from the underlying muscle, leaving the pectoral fascia behind. Volkmann clearly described the extirpation of the axillary mass.[229]

Billroth also removed the whole breast, although he was not convinced that a careful local extirpation of small tumours together with a fair amount of surrounding textures would not serve the purpose just as well. He excised the pectoral fascia together with a substantial layer of the underlying muscle only in the case of adherence.

After the removal of the specimen, he carefully inspected the woundbed for fragments of the tumour. After all bleeding had been arrested, the skin incision was lengthened and any enlarged or hardened nodes were digitally removed, together with the axillary fat. The axillary vein was, as a rule, exposed.[230]

Since the introduction of antiseptic wound treatment in 1877, the operative mortality of mastectomies with removal of axillary nodes had dropped from 21.3 to 10.5 per cent and the overall mortality from 15.7 to 5.8 percent.[231] Billroth belonged to those who had adopted an initial attitude of reserve towards Lister's innovation.

In the same year in which Billroth's well-known book on diseases of the breast appeared, 1880, Samuel Weissel Gross (1837–89), lecturer in clinical surgery at The Jefferson Medical College Hospital in Philadelphia (this institute apparently played a leading role at the time in the United States), reported on the results of surgical treatment of over 200 cases of breast cancer. Gross had treated the first 55 by incomplete eradication, without having cleared out the axilla in any systematic way: these patients had all died from recurrences shortly after the operation. After he had proceeded to complete excision of the mamma with removal of the pectoral fascia and systematic extirpation of the axillar mass, he could boast of a three years survival rate of 19.44 per cent.[232]

Removal of the axillary fat in all cases was also recommended in 1883 by professor Ernst Georg Ferdinand Küster (1839–after 1922), at the time chief surgeon at the Augusta-Spital in Berlin. Ever since that method had become a routine procedure, he had observed but one instance occurring in the axilla amongst 95 cases of recurrence. Six years later, his assistant, Lothar Heidenhain (1860–1940), demonstrated in operative specimens that, in many cases, the pectoral fascia is very thin. When separating the fascia from the muscle, connective tissue fragments and glandular remnants can therefore stay behind. There are, furthermore, lymphatics alongside the blood vessels running in the retromammary connective tissue from the lacteal gland to the fascia. In two-thirds of the cases of breast cancer, numerous small metastases are found within these lymph vessels. They soon penetrate into the fascia and then follow delicate protrusions of that structure into the muscle.[233] In the ten years that had passed since Billroth had published his microscopic descriptions, histological techniques had made great advances. Thus Heidenhain — whose father was a renowned professor of physiology and microscopical anatomy in Breslau at the time — had at his disposal modern fixation and staining techniques using celloidin and haematoxylin, as well as the microtome. His paper attracted much attention at the time. Modern studies, however, do not seem to have confirmed Heidenhain's observations, since no direct lymphatic routes between the breast and the pectoralis major muscle are shown in Haagensen's diagram of the lymphatic drainage of the breast.[234] As long as the tumour is still freely movable over the underlayer, the muscle is usually still healthy, Heidenhain declared. It only becomes involved when a metastatic deposit develops over the fascia or, by contiguity, the tumour itself penetrates between its fibres. With reference to surgical treatment, Heidenhain concluded that a coherent layer of the entire muscle surface should also be removed if the tumour is still movable. Should, however, the tumour be fixed to the chest wall, the pectoralis major muscle should be completely removed, including the connective tissue behind it.[235]

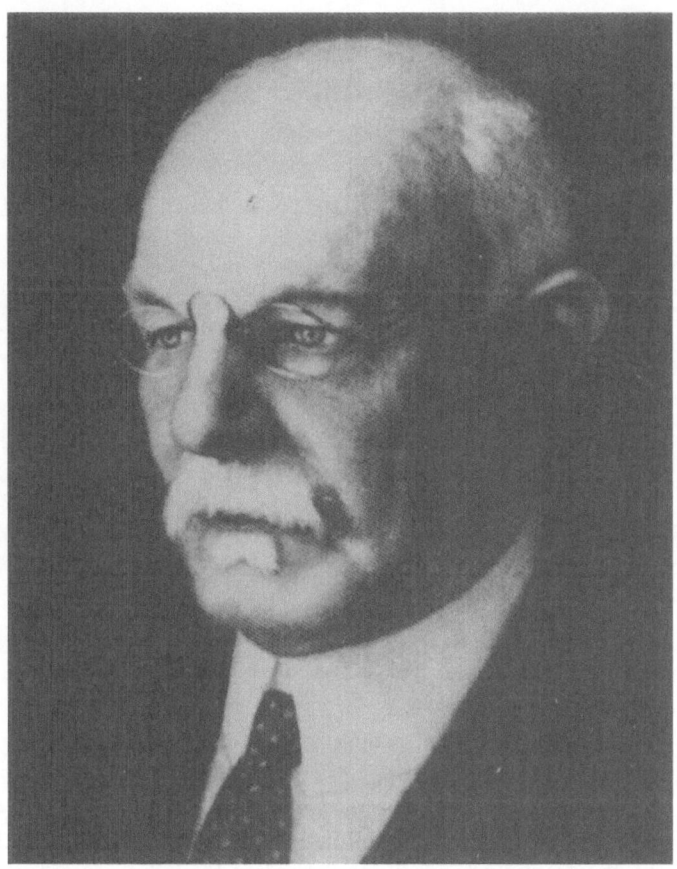

Fig. 33. William Steward Halsted.

In 1882, William Steward Halsted (1852–1922) (Fig. 33), working in The Roosevelt Hospital in New York, started to remove the pectoralis muscle as a matter of routine. He reported briefly on it in 1890 and once again, but this time more elaborately, in 1894. By that time, Halsted was professor of surgery at the newly formed College of Medicine at Johns Hopkins University in Baltimore. In the Welch Medical Library of that university, a famous picture by John Singer Sargent represents Halsted in academic attire in the company of the pathologist William H. Welch, the internist William Osler and the gynaecologist Howard A. Kelly. These were the 'Four Doctors' who, as first members of the Johns Hopkins medical faculty, placed the teaching of medicine in the United States on a modern basis by, amongst other things, uniting the education of physicians with the training of medical scientists, in which a good deal of prominence was given to the laboratory. In treating breast cancer, Halsted recommended that 'the suspected tissues should be removed in one piece lest the wound become infected by the division of tissue invaded by the disease, or by division of the lymphatic vessels containing cancer cells, and because shreds or pieces of cancerous

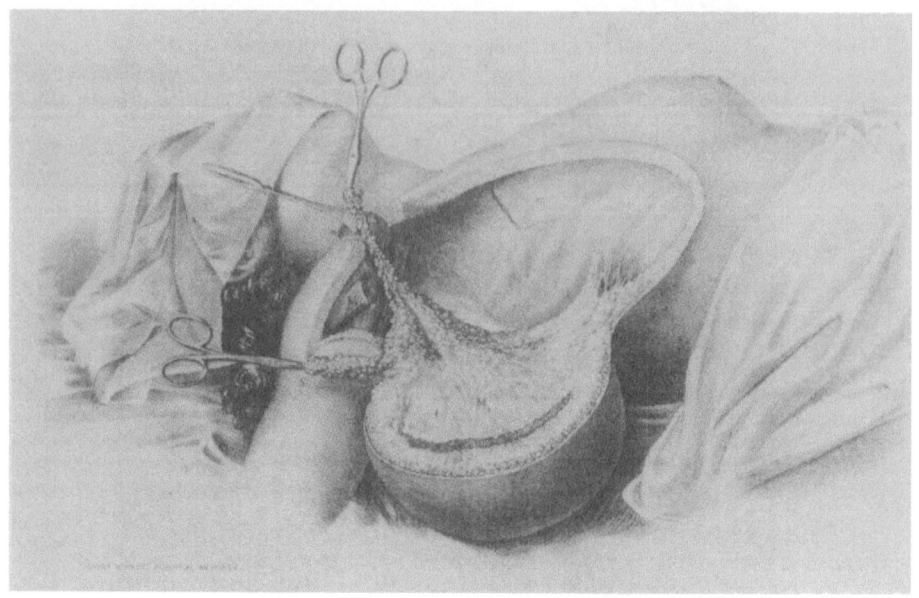

Fig. 34.   Diagram showing Halsted's operation.

tissue might be readily overlooked in a piecemeal extirpation'[236] (Fig. 34). Only ten days after Halsted's 1894 paper was published, Willy Meyer (1854–1932), a German-born surgeon at the New York Graduate School of Medicine, described a technique which was very similar to that of Halsted, the only essential difference being that Meyer removed both pectoral muscles.[237] Radical mastectomy had reached its final form.

American surgery was at the time strongly orientated towards Germany and Austria and many Americans were making study trips to the Old Continent. Halsted too, had been across the Atlantic. When called to the chair of surgery at Johns Hopkins, he founded a school of surgery which was reminiscent of Billroth's school in Vienna. In his first publication in 1890/91, he gave evidence of being familiar with Volkmann's operation. In his subsequent work he quoted many more German surgeons: Bergmann, Billroth, Czerny, Fischer, Güssenbauer, König, Küster and Lücke, but he referred nowhere to the fundamental work of Charles H. Moore, which we discussed briefly. Nor did he seem to be aware of Mitchell Banks' papers, read in 1877, 1882 and 1887, respectively, to various medical societies in Great Britain, in which he advocated the removal of the breast 'and the glands all away in one piece'. Banks (b. 1842), who was surgeon to the Liverpool Royal Infirmary and lecturer on anatomy at the school of anatomy, published his views in the *Liverpool and Manchester Surgical Reports* for 1878, and once again in the *Liverpool medico-chirurgical Journal* in 1883. Since these journals had only a limited circulation, Banks' proposition attracted little attention, even in his own country and none at all abroad.[238]

Scientific materialism, which since the middle of the last century has governed medical thinking to a high degree, also stimulated the critical faculty. 'The main task of our time is criticism', Billroth once stated, 'and going with it are knowledge, experience and quiet'. During his time at Zürich he started to publish annual reports which not only offered crude figures, but also a critical evaluation of the cases treated. Other surgical clinics followed suit and such annual reports are an extremely valuable source of information for the student of nineteenth-century surgery. Another typical product of that period was the statistical review of one particular disease over a certain period. An outstanding early example was the statistical study of cancer, published by Winiwarter in 1878 and already referred to in Chapter 8.[212] It comprised 170 cases of breast cancer seen by his preceptor professor Billroth in Zürich and in Vienna, between 1867 and 1875. At the time of publication, 19 patients (13.3%) out of 143 who had undergone surgery, were alive and supposed to be free of disease for at least three years, or had died from other causes. Since, in the period under review, antiseptic wound treatment had not yet been introduced in Billroth's department, we are not too surprised to find that operative mortality was as high as 23.7 per cent.

Winiwarter's report still makes good reading. With regard to aetiology we find that solitary trauma, which for many centuries had been looked upon as a major cause, now gained little credence, although Winiwarter was inclined to allow some importance to recurrent injuries. Age, married status, parity, occurrence in relation to benign lesions, heredity, clinical signs, localization in various parts of the breast, metastasis, duration of symptoms prior to surgery, length of survival, operative results with and without removal of axillary glands, postoperative complications – from which we gain a good impression of the horrors of pre-antiseptic surgery – were all thoroughly discussed and supported by figures.

In the same year 1878, a similar report on 229 cases, operated on between 1850 and 1878, was issued from the department of Friedrich von Esmarch (1823–1908) in Kiel. This gave a three-year survival rate of 11.7 per cent. It was customary at the time to accept a reporting interval of three years, relying on a statement by Volkmann that if careful examination failed to detect local recurrence of regional or distant metastasis after one year, hope of survival might be entertained. After two years one could be almost certain; after three years survival was the rule almost without exception. The fact that survival rates were being presented at all, shows that, during the decades which had elapsed since Velpeau stated that most patients were lost sight of after their operations, post-operative follow-up had become an accepted procedure.

William H. Cooper from the Department of Surgery of the New York Hospital and Cornell Medical College tabulated the three-year survival results of a number of – mainly German – clinics[239] (Table 1). Such summary lists should be viewed with reserve. Johannes Adrianus Korteweg (1851–1930) in The Netherlands, professor of surgery in Groningen, Amsterdam and Leyden successively between 1880 and 1903, critically reviewed the cancer statistics of the last three decades of the nineteenth century in a number of articles which gained him a certain reputation at home and abroad.[240] Such returns are, he explained, not mutually comparable, if for no other

Table 1.

Type of operation	Author	Year	No. of cases	% 3 year cures
1. Partial or complete mastectomy, whether or not with removal of pectoral fascia and axillary nodes	Winiwarter (Billroth)	1867–1875	143	4.7 *Average: 4.7*
2. Complete mastectomy and axillary dissection in majority of cases	Oldekop (Esmarch, Kiel)	1850–1878	220	11.7
	Dietrich (Lücke, Strassburg)	1872–1890	148	16.2
	Horner (Krönlein, Zürich)	1881–1893	144	19.4
	Poulsen (Copenhagen)	1870–1888	110	20
	Banks (Liverpool)	1877	46	20
	Schmid (Küster, Berlin)	1871–1885	228	21.5 *Average: 18.1*
3. Complete mastectomy, axillary dissection, removal of pectoral fascia and greater or lesser amounts of pectoral muscle	Sprengel (Volkmann, Halle)	1874–1878	200	11
	Schmidt (Czerny, Heidelberg)	1877–1886	112	18.8
	Rotter (Bergmann, Berlin)		30	20
	Mahler (Czerny, Heidelberg)	1887–1897	150	21
	Joerss (Helferich, Greifswald)	1885–1893	98	28.5 *Average: 19.9*
4. Modern radical mastectomy	Halsted	1889–1894	76	45
	Halsted	1907	232	38.3

Modified after William A. Cooper.

reason than that widely differing operative approaches were used. This certainly applies to the authors listed in Cooper's second and third horizontal column and, in addition, one surgeon would be prepared to wield the knife whereas another would abstain from active treatment. Korteweg also pointed out that older statistics dated back to pre-antiseptic times and these, understandably, showed a much higher operative mortality. On the other hand, there were probably less instances of local recurrences then, than after the introduction of antisepsis. The preference for primary wound healing could induce surgeons to cut away less skin than before. Von Esmarch, for instance, always removed all skin of the breast together with the tumour, irrespective of its size, being satisfied with a healing by second intention. Korteweg was, moreover, struck by the paradox which appeared in pre-antiseptic statistics in particular, that the outlook for tumours, which had existed for a long time before they were operated on, was often better than that for lesions which had been recently noticed for the first time. On this observation he based his proposition that there are two varieties of breast cancer, a relatively benign and a relatively malignant variety, and that we are, on principle, only able to cure the former. The three-year survival rate of patients without axillary indurations appeared to be twice as high as that of those who showed enlarged nodes at the time of operation.

Korteweg expressed the opinion that, with the methods of treatment used at the turn of the century, no further improvement of curative results was to be expected.[241]

CHAPTER 10

The twentieth century

Centennial years were seldom real milestones in the history of medicine. The expiration of the nineteenth century, however, marked the conclusion of a most memorable period, characterized by the rise of scientific materialism, with internationally accepted methods of research and principles of judgements. In the field of oncology, of mammary carcinoma in particular, very important strides forward had been made with regard to the morphology of tumours. The very word 'morphology' dates, in fact, from the nineteenth century since it first appeared in print in 1800, having been coined by Goethe.[242] The golden harvest of the last few decades was embodied in a superb book with a companion microscopical atlas entitled *Die Lehre von den Geschwülsten* by Max Borst (1869–1946), who was assistant to the Department of Pathology of the University of Würzburg.[243]

Among the different pathogenetic views on cancer advanced in the nineteenth century, the embryonic theory in particular continued, for quite a while, to have a following in our own century. It was upheld by, amongst others, the distinguished pathologist professor Hugo Ribbert in Bonn. In his books on malignant neoplasia in man, which may be counted amongst the best to appear shortly before the First World War, Ribbert emphasized that malignant tumours have their own independent manner of growth and do not increase in size on account of progressive changes in adjacent cell groups, as was believed by some.[244]

Another view that persisted for many years was that carcinoma, once it was established, behaved like a kind of parasite. This was upheld by James Ewing (1866–1943), professor of pathology at Cornell University, Ithaca, and by many others. The tumour only depended on its host for its blood supply, but otherwise acted quite autonomously. This parasitic conception of cancer was only to be abandoned in the forties, mainly because of the work of Charles Huggins and his collaborators, whom we shall discuss later.

Fairly recently, it became clear that the unicentric, single-focus one-cell or two-cell origin of cancer is no longer tenable. Particularly characteristic of cancer of the breast — and of the skin, pancreas, prostate and gastrointestinal tract — is a multicentric origin.[245]

The notion that breast carcinoma was initially a local disease, once it became generally accepted in the latter half of the nineteenth century, had encouraged the operative approach to the disease. Shortly before the end of the century, radical mastectomy had become a standard procedure and there were even reports of first attempts at supraradical interventions.

The very fact that supraradical procedures were being tried at all illustrates that the Halsted operation, in spite of being superior to any other technique proposed up till that time, did not offer a basic extension of operability as such. The realization that surgery could never be the final answer to all cases of cancer, as well as the failure to detect a causative living germ in spite of intensive research, cast the first serious damper on the scientific optimism which had marked Western medicine since the first spectacular triumphs of bacteriology and surgery.

Cancer is receiving more and more attention, wrote Churchill in 1888.[217] In 1895, the first specialized medical journal, the *Revue des maladies cancéreuses*, made its appearance in Paris. After only five years, however, it disappeared from the scene, owing to insufficient active support on the part of the profession.[246] It did not take long, however, for new journals to come out. In 1903, the *Zeitschrift für Krebsforschung* was started in Germany by the 'Zentralkomitee zur Erforschung und Bekämpfung der Krebskrankheit', which was established in 1900. The *Reports of the Imperial Cancer Research Fund* in Great-Britain were first issued in 1904, the *Bulletin de l'Association française pour l'Etude du Cancer* in 1908 and many others were to follow in the subsequent years.[247] In contrast to the ill-fated *Revue des maladies cancéreuses*, these later journals were supported by substantial organizations. The establishment of many such organizations all over the world in the early twentieth century confirms Churchill's statement.

The knowledge that was gained about breast cancer during the first three-quarters of the present century had been laboriously acquired in three different, though entwined ways: by epidemiological studies, by laboratory research and by practical experience with several types of treatment. We will conduct our survey accordingly.

EPIDEMIOLOGY AND STATISTICS

An early contribution to the epidemiology of breast cancer was made by T.H.C. Stevenson in 1915, who in an *Annual Report of the Registrar-General of Births, Deaths and Marriages in England and Wales*, drew attention to the fact that, after the age of forty-five, the mortality rate for breast cancer was markedly higher for single than for married women.[248] This confirmed the observation made by several seventeenth- and eighteenth-century authors, that there were a relatively large number of nuns amongst breast cancer patients.

The first modern case-control study on breast cancer was carried out − also in Great-Britain − by Janet Elizabeth Lane-Claypon (b. 1877) in 1926.[249] On comparing a series of 508 breast cancer patients from London with a group of 509 healthy women, she found that cancer patients had married later, were of a lower parity, had breast-fed their babies less often, and, on average, had a longer menstrual life. She found, moreover, an increased family risk and noted that no less than 28.6 per cent of cancer patients attributed their disease to antecedent breast injury. Petrakis has recently pointed out that the case-control technique which was employed by

Mrs. Lane-Claypoᵗ has subsequently been applied by many others and is still in common use in eᵖidemiologic studies. Her work, therefore, truly represents a historic milestone. Her first report, in which she presented a retrospective study on the results of operative treatment, will be dealt with below.

The clinical features demonstrated by Lane-Claypon were, on the whole, confirmed in a great many subsequent studies. In more recent times, when women were less inclined to breast-feed children, the non-lactation factor gave rise to conflicting reports. It was also by means of epidemiologic studies that the existence of ethnic differences was discovered. An early example is the study carried out in 1929 by Herbert L. Lombard and Carl R. Doering amongst the foreign-born population in Massachusetts: they found a low breast cancer rate among Italian and Russian women.[248]

Time and again attention has been paid during the last half century to the natural survival rates of patients with untreated breast cancer. Such data are of course not without significance since the result of treatment is expressed in duration of survival. It appeared from the different reports that the average duration of life after the onset of symptoms was about 38 months. Of course, the survival period of individual patients varied greatly. In 1962, Bloom, Richardson and Harries discussed the most important articles on the subject.[250] Table 2, borrowed from their paper, summarizes the survival rates in years, as presented by various authors. Their article provides a special flavour for the historian, however, because of the fact that these authors had the opportunity of studying the records of 250 patients who died from untreated breast cancer in the Cancer Charity Wards of the Middlesex Hospital in London between 1805 – when the first cancer case was admitted – and 1933. No less than 68 per cent of these women had ulcerating tumours when they presented themselves. Figure 35 is their graphic presentation of the survival rate of the Middlesex cases, plotted for comparison with that of the 'natural' survival rate of a healthy female population of similar age distribution. After 173 years, John Howard's expectation, expressed in 1791 in his letter to the Directors of The Middlesex Hospital, that the permanent presence of cancer patients would provide ample opportunity for studying the natural history of the disease, was fulfilled!

An intriguing statistical observation was made by Clemens von Pirquet (1874–1929), the well-known Viennese paediatrician and founder of the science of allergy,

Table 2. Untreated breast cancer. Survival rates from onset of symptoms (various authors)

Author	No. of cases	Survival rate in years (%)			
		3	5	10	15
Greenwood (1926)	651	34	16	–	–
Daland (1927)	100	–	22	5	0
Nathanson and Welch (1936)*	100	40	18	5	0
Forber (1931)	64	30	17	–	–
Present series	250	44	18	3.6	0.8

*Survival rates obtained from graph.
After HJG Bloom et al.[250]

90

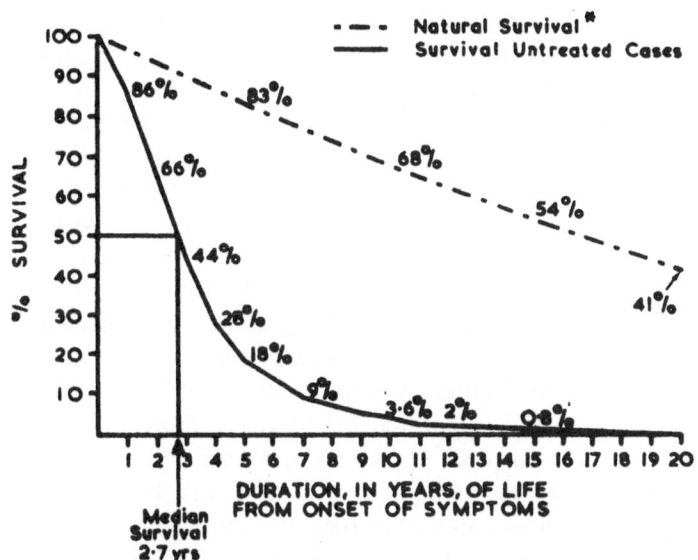

Fig. 35. Survival of untreated breast cancer. Middlesex Hospital, 1805–1933.

when he found a bi-modal age distribution of patients with mammary cancer. One peak represented the patients who were 45 to 49 years of age, when the diagnosis was first made, the second peak was at about 65 years. This observation has since been confirmed by several cancer statisticians in Europe and in the United States. The phenomenon was studied by F. de Waard and his associates in Utrecht in 1960 and 1964. Proceeding from the assumption that oestrogen plays an important part in the formation of breast cancer, they took account of ovarian oestrogen disturbance and, alternatively, of adrenocortical oestrogen disturbance. Dividing a given breast cancer population into two groups, on the basis of the presence or absence of certain signs suggestive of adrenal oestrogen production – obesity, hypertension and decreased glucose tolerance –, they found that the second – postmenopausal – statistical age peak was made up of patients showing signs of imbalance in adrenal oestrogen. They concluded, in addition, that a heredity tendency existed in this group which was absent in the other.[251] Statistical analysis, of course, plays a prominent part in the evaluation of different types of treatment – innumerable evaluations of this kind have appeared ever since the early twenties.

LABORATORY RESEARCH

Microscopic cancer research, already begun in the early nineteenth century, was energetically continued in our own age. Since the twenties, many pathologists have been looking for histological features which might be indicative of the intrinsic malignity of individual tumours. The degree of tubular differentiation, the staining of nuclei, the frequency of hyperchromatic and mitotic figures have been taken into account. Bloom held that a combined classification, using clinical stage and histologic grade,

91

would provide a more accurate guide to prognosis than either factor alone.[252] It appeared, however, that in the majority of cases the prognostic accuracy of histological grading of breast cancer is questionable.[253]

The major trend in the twentieth century, as compared to the more static anatomical and microscopical studies of the nineteenth, has been towards an experimental approach of the cancer problem. Basic research into the genesis and the biology of breast cancer was seriously hampered by the fact that this disease was not easily modelled in the laboratory animal. The first attempts at producing cancer in an experimental animal were made by Arthur Nathan Hanau (1858–1900), a reader of pathology and pathologic anatomy in Zürich, by means of transplantation. In 1889, he grafted fragments of a spontaneous vulvar carcinoma of a rat into the scrotum of two male rats. After six weeks these two animals died and Hanau found proliferations along their vasa deferentia and a carcinosis of the peritoneum in both cases. By implanting some of the material in yet another animal, he once again obtained peritoneal carcinosis. On microscopic examination, the tumour was a cornified epithelial carcinoma. Although these experiments were performed in the very period when cancer research meant the hunt for a living agent, Hanau was careful not to present his findings as evidence of a parasitic origin of cancer, but as the outcome of the transplantation of live tumour cells.[254] Hanau's pioneer work in experimental oncology was largely ignored and he took his own life in August 1900, it was said from sheer frustration, but he was suffering from cancer and did not want to wait events.

At the turn of the century, transplantation experiments came to the fore. A truly remarkable observation was reported to the venerable Academy of Science in Paris by M. Bra in 1899. He had been successful, so he claimed, in transplanting human cancer into trees. After six months, these trees were showing cancer-like outgrowths. One elm even developed a general 'cancrosis', with ulcers appearing in the bark. When rabbits were fed with seeds from that tree, they developed round ulcers of the stomach.[255] The reaction of the members of the Academy is not known. Jakob Wolff, when summarizing this report in his book in 1906, limited himself to the cautious remark that it had not as yet been confirmed by others.

The question remained whether successful transplantations were to be regarded as indications of the parasitogenic origin of tumours or merely as tissue grafts. Of paramount importance in this connection were the experiments reported in 1903 by the Danish veterinarian, bacteriologist and pathologist Carl Oluf Jensen, which we mentioned in Chapter 7.[200] Shortly afterwards, E.F. Bashford and J.A. Murray, working on tumour resistance of the host animal in the recently established London laboratory of the Imperial Cancer Research Fund, greatly contributed to the general acceptance of mouse mammary carcinoma as a standard experimental research tool.[256] The mouse became still more useful as an experimental animal for cancer research, since it became possible to produce, by selective breeding, strains either quite resistant or particularly susceptible to cancer. This was first achieved in Chicago by Maud Slye (b. 1879), who, between 1914 and 1928, wrote a number of important papers on the subject of cancer and heredity, and who showed, in 1915, that in mice resistance to cancer is a Mendelian dominant factor and susceptibility a recessive one.[257] In 1910,

Ernst Freund (1863–1943) and Gisa Kaminer (1883–1941), working in the 'Rudolf-Stiftung' in Vienna, developed a diagnostic serum reaction. This was based on their observation that in the blood serum of healthy people cancer cells are destroyed by a 'normal-acid', whereas they remain intact in the serum of cancer patients.[258] This reaction was not frequently applied in cases of breast cancer, as far as I know. But when the originators renewed the subject in 1924, considering their discovery to be a manifestation of a somatic disposition, they contributed highly to the revival of interest in the phenomenon of 'host response', which occurred in the twenties.

The experimental production of tar cancer in rabbits by the Japanese research workers Katsusaburo Yamagiwa (1863–1930) and Kokichi Ichikawa (b. 1887) in 1916,[259] and the discovery of the carcinogenic properties of dibenzanthracene compounds by James Wilfred Cook (b. 1900) and his collaborators in 1932, established that, in a general sense, cancer can be the outcome of prolonged chemical stimulation.[260] The carcinogenic effects of a number of physical agents were known to exist long before the turn of the century; for example, sunlight on the skin of the face, pressure of a pipe stem on the lower lip and chronic irritation of the tongue by decayed and dirty teeth. The danger of ionizing rays was realized in the early years of this century and was affirmed most spectacularly by the consequences of the atomic bomb explosions, which put an end to the Second World War. The suspicion that physical trauma plays a part in the origin of breast cancer is probably as old as medicine itself.

In 1939, Georgina May Bonser and J.W. Orr were able to induce mammary cancer in mice, using polycyclic hydrocarbons.[261] Much experimental work has since been done on the ability of several chemical compounds to produce breast cancer.

The ancient conception that the cyclic changes, which take place in the tissues of the breast and the mucous membrane of the uterus, are carcinogenic stimuli was once more voiced in 1922 by Bernhard Fischer-Wasels (b. 1877) in Frankfurt am Main.[262]

An American pathologist, Francis Peyton Rous (1879–1970), who was attached to the Rockefeller Institute for Medical Research in New York for the greater part of his life, added fresh fuel to the nineteenth-century suspicion that malignant processes are aroused by life germs. In 1910, he demonstrated the transferability of fowl sarcoma by injecting filtered extracts.[263] Later, Rous and his collaborators discovered several other chicken tumours, each caused by a distinctive virus.[264] The existence of virogenetic tumours was a controversial issue for years. In 1936, John Joseph Bittner (1904–1961) in Bar Harbor, Maine, found that breast cancer in mice was transmitted by a factor present in the milk of the mother-animal. It soon became apparent that this 'milk-factor' was a virus.[265] Important work on this subject was also done by Remmert Korteweg (1884–1961) in Amsterdam. In the seventies, the search for a human mammary tumour virus was rigorously pursued.

In 1966, Rous received the Nobel prize for his work in the field of tumour viruses. This was his well-earned reward for having disregarded the warning, once given to him by his Baltimore teacher William H. Welch, not to stake his scientific career on so precarious an endeavour as cancer research.

Rous' co-recipient of the prize was Charles Brenton Huggins (b. 1901) of the

University of Chicago. Huggins was given the award on account of his work on the influence of hormones on certain tumours of man. His ideas on hormone dependency 'far transcends its practical applications', Rous said when discussing the implication of Huggins' work, 'for it means that thought and endeavor in cancer research has been misdirected in consequence of the belief that tumour cells are anarchic'.[266]

Huggins' research familiarized the scientific world with the basic concept of the 'hormone-dependence' of some types of malignant neoplasia. The influence of hormones on the development of breast cancer was suggested by the work of A.E.C. Lathrop and that of Leo Loeb (1869–1959), in St. Louis, who, in 1916, found that the incidence of breast cancer could be reduced by removing the ovaries in mice of a strain in which this disease occurred frequently.[267] This observation was affirmed in 1927 by the Czech-born Carol Ferdinand Cori (b. 1896), who was working at that time at the State Institute for the Study of Malignant Diseases in Buffalo. He established that early removal of ovaries in mice of a dominant cancer strain prevented the development of spontaneous adenocarcinoma in all cases.[268] In 1935 Antoine-Marcellin Lacassagne (1884–1971) of the Radium Institute of the University of Paris, showed that, by contrast, injections of oestrogen caused adenocarcinoma of the breast in mice.[269] After the Second World War, outstanding work on hormone dependant mouse tumours was done by Otto Frits Ernst Mühlbock (1906–1979) and his group in The Netherlands Cancer Institute in Amsterdam.

SEVERAL TYPES OF TREATMENT

With the intention of giving the reader an impression of how different types of therapy have contributed to our present knowledge of breast cancer and to our practical approach to that disease, we will now trace in brief the development in our century of surgery, radiation therapy, hormonal treatment and chemotherapy respectively.

Surgery

Soon after Halsted and Meyer had described their radical operation, Rudolph Matas (1860–1957) in New Orleans, who is mainly remembered for his pioneer contributions in the field of vasular surgery, and several others pointed out that this operation could make no pretence to being complete. For extensive as it was, it left the supraclavicular and the internal mammary nodes alone. Matas referred in his argumentation to the beautifully illustrated standard work, entitled *Anatomie, physiologie, pathologie des vaisseaux lymphatiques* (Paris, 1874) by Marie-Philibert-Constant Sappey (1810–96), one of the best French anatomists of the nineteenth century.[270] The validity of the objection could not be contested and even before the turn of the century a few surgeons, amongst whom Halsted himself and C.W.J. Westerman in the Dutch town of Haarlem, made attempts to meet the requirements of radicality more closely by removing the supraclavicular nodes. Halsted himself claimed, in 1907, to have 'cleaned out' the supraclavicular region in 119 patients. Only two of the 44 patients, in whom the supraclavicular nodes were found to contain metastatic deposits, were alive and well after five years.[271] Westerman reported, in 1910, on a case of local recurrence, in which he had exarticulated the arm and resected three ribs, covering the thoracic wall defect with a pedicled flap left over from the amputation. In two other patients, he had performed a partial thoracic wall excision and closed the defect with the remaining healthy breast.[272] This was done at a time when anaesthesia consisted of ether or chloroform being dripped onto a frame-mask by a surgical resident or a nurse, when blood transfusion was hardly practised at all, when intravenous administration of other fluids was not yet heard of and when ligature was the only means to arrest haemorrhage. Westerman's first patient was alive and well after $1\frac{1}{2}$ years, the other two died within some months and several weeks, respectively. After a few years such supraradical operations were abandoned when they appeared to increase the operative mortality without improving the survival rate.

Halsted's original operation, however, was soon popular all over the world. A majority of surgeons felt that, given the particular anatomy of the region, it meant an optimal attainment at an acceptable operative risk. It reduced, for one thing, the rate of local recurrences and it was expected that it would also better the survival rate.

In 1924, Mrs. Lane-Claypon presented the first of her two important statistical surveys of breast cancer. This contained a retrospective study of 20,000 operations collected from the medical literature of the past twenty-five years. For those patients who underwent a radical mastectomy, she calculated a survival of 43.2% after three years and 33.1% after five years. Women who had been treated with a non-radical operation had a three-year survival rate of only 29.2%.[273]

Across the Atlantic, William Crawford White reported, in 1927, on 157 radical mastectomies performed in the Roosevelt Hospital in New York. After five years, 36 per cent of the patients was alive and in good health, and after ten years, this percentage was 24.[274] In the twenties the reporting interval appears to have been tacitly extended from three to five years or even more, a yard-stick already used by a few centres — the Massachusetts General Hospital, for instance — in the early years of this century.

Relatively favourable reports, like the two cited above, no doubt helped to strengthen the confidence of the surgical profession in the Halsted operation. Indeed, for some thirty years or more since the turn of the century, there was little doubt as to the justification of that standard operation. Thus, these few decades constitute the only period in the history of breast cancer in which some degree of therapeutic consensus existed. Even today, Halsted's operation is by no means outdated. Haagensen, working in the Columbia-Presbyterian Medical Center in New York, can be cited as a prominent recent champion (Fig. 36).

Lane-Claypon, as well as White, pointed out that the postoperative prognosis after a complete operation is related to the stage of the disease at the moment of operation. White stated that the overall five-year tumour-free survival rate of operable cases amounted to 30 or 35 per cent at the time, but that it was twice as high — 60 to 65 per cent — in the absence of enlarged axillary nodes. Nineteenth-century returns had shown the same 2:1 ratio of survival in favour of cases without axillary involvement.[275] It is true that at that time the accepted reporting time was only three years.

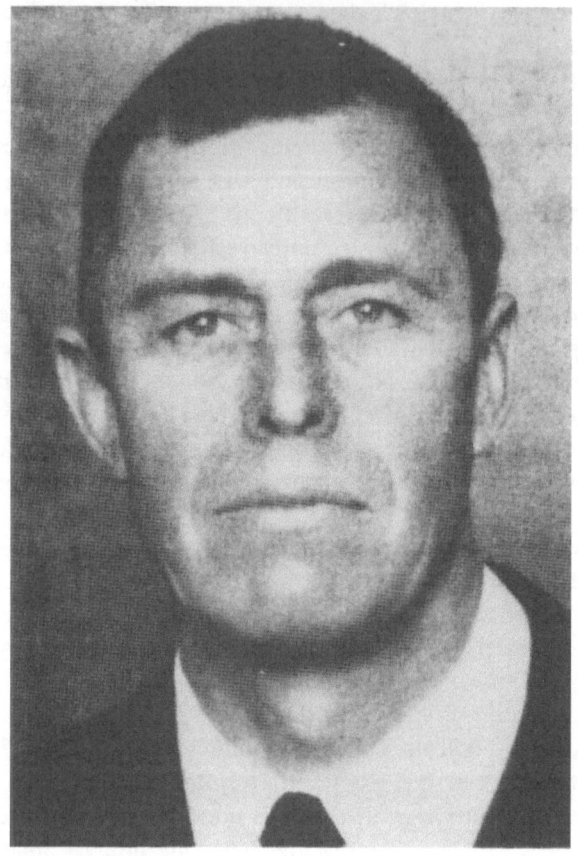

Fig. 36.   Cushman Davies Haagensen.

Korteweg repeatedly pointed out that the data presented in the statistical reports published by clinics in the nineteenth century hardly admitted reliable comparison because, amongst other things, divergent and non-specified criteria were being applied in assessing operability. Carl Steinthal (b. 1859) concluded, after an analysis of the results of breast cancer surgery in the municipal Katharinen-hospital in Stuttgart, Germany, that different clinical types offered a different prospect of curability. On the basis of his retrospective findings, he drew up a clinical classification in three stages, conducive to a prospective evaluation of patients with regard to operability and prognosis:

Stage I : small-sized, slowly growing tumour, no adherence, axillary nodes absent or only apparent at operation;
Stage II : obviously enlarging, adherence to the skin, axillary nodes;
Stage III: large tumour adherent to skin and underlying structures, enlargement of axillary and supraclavicular nodes.

Since none of Steinthal's patients belonging to the last group had survived the operation for any length of time, stage III henceforth meant inoperability.[276]

Steinthal's staging, which, after its introduction in 1905, was widely used for many years in Europe in particular, has been succeeded by ever more refined systems in which the features of the tumour itself, as well as regional and distant metastasis are accounted for. It does not serve any purpose to enumerate them here: surgical readers will be familiar with some of these classifications and a survey of the most important ones can be found in Mansfield.

The older classifications have been devised by individual surgeons or centres, the more recent ones by national or even international committees. This is a reflection of the increasing scale on which cancer research is being organised.

It is not always possible, however, to make an accurate assessment of distant or even regional metastases by means of physical examination alone. As a rule, the infraclavicular nodes in the apical area of the axilla, as well as the internal mammary nodes, escape detection by palpation. In view of the grave prognostic significance of metastases in these nodes, Haagensen, in 1955, began to perform preliminary biopsy of the apex of the axilla, combined with biopsy of the internal mammary nodes when-ever any doubt existed regarding the extent of regional spread in seemingly operable cases.[277] In the same year, E.A. van Slooten in Amsterdam independently devised the same procedure.

The importance of the internal mammary lymphatic chain as a route of dissemi-nation was realized only comparatively recently, although Petrus Camper had des-cribed and depicted internal mammary 'mossy glands' of the inner side of the sternum in relation to breast cancer as early as 1779[278] (Fig. 17). It was only in 1927 that William Simpson Handley (1872–1962) of the Middlesex Hospital once more called attention to these structures, expressing his belief that they are frequently, if not always, involved by the time the axillary nodes are enlarged. He claimed to have removed the internal mammary nodes 'on several occasions' at the completion of radical mastectomy.[279]

After the Second World War, Handley's example was followed by a number of surgeons, amongst whom his son Richard Handley, who succeeded him at the Middlesex Hospital, M. Margottini and Pietro Bacalossi in Rome and Milan, E. Dahl-Iversen in Copenhagen, Jerome A. Urban in England and Owen Harding Wangensteen (1898–1981), surgeon to the University of Minnesota Hospital. After the war these surgeons practised and advocated a 'supra-radical' mastectomy, in which they extended the operative field into the mediastinum and into the neck.[280]

J. Englebert Dunphy (b. 1908), professor of surgery at Harvard Medical School, Boston, when discussing the place of surgery in the treatment of cancer in 1953, concluded that there was no evidence at the time to justify any general or routine extension of the established operations for cancer. 'The consistently similar results of well performed surgery of the breast, stomach, colon and rectum over the years in the hands of different surgeons (for example, . . . 50 per cent survival in cancer of the breast . . .) suggests that this represents about the number of tumors biologically susceptible to surgical extirpation'.[245] The opinion that biologic predeterminism is the most important factor influencing prognosis, was also expressed by Ian Macdonald at the University of Southern California School of Medicine[253] and by several others.

The selfsame 1920's, in which expansive tendencies set in, also witnessed the rise of a diametrically opposed trend aimed at a reduction in scope of the operation, while applying radiation as a peremptory supplementary treatment. The evolutions of this particular course will be outlined in the next section. After the Second World War, when it appeared that the results of radical mastectomy were not upon re-examination, as good as had generally been supposed, the value of the Halsted operation became seriously challenged. This resulted, among some clinicians, in a somewhat nihilistic attitude towards the treatment of breast cancer in general. It induced others, like Haagensen, to adopt more rigid criteria for the operation.[281]

Radiation therapy

The limitations of cancer surgery were always an inducement to look for other modes of therapy. It did not take long after the discovery of X-rays in 1895 by Wilhelm Conrad Röntgen (1845–1923) in Würzburg, before their possible action on malignant tumours became the subject of investigation.

As early as 1896 Hermann Gocht (1869–1938) (Fig. 37), at the time an assistant at the surgical department of Hermann Kümmell in the Neue Allgemeine Krankenhaus in Hamburg, tried the new rays in two cases of mammary cancer. He published his findings in the very first issue of the first journal exclusively devoted to the medical use of X-rays, the *Fortschritte auf dem Gebiete der Roentgenstrahlen*. One patient was suffering from an ulcerating process and the other had a recurrence with axillary nodes after repeated operations. In both cases the pain disappeared. The first patient died on the seventeenth day of treatment from cachexy and sepsis, after repeated profuse haemorrhages from her ulcer. The second woman expired after three months, in which time her swellings had only increased in size. For reasons of economy Gocht had made use of tubes, which were no longer serviceable for photographic purposes. The voltage was rather high, he wrote, it amounted to 50 volts at least. The tube was placed at a distance of six or seven centimetres and the frequency of the sessions was 15 to 30 minutes twice a day. The surroundings were protected with flexible lead.[282]

In the same year, 1896, Emile Herman Grubbé (1875–1960) in Chicago treated a patient with a large, ulcerating mammary cancer in a similar way, but the patient died within a month.[283]

Another early pioneer in this field was Georg Clemens Perthes (1869–1927), professor of surgery in Leipzig, who is particularly remembered for his test for varicose veins and for his description of juvenile osteochondrosis of the hip which have both become eponymous in the medical profession. In 1903 he ascribed the curative effect of X-rays to inhibition of cell division.[284]

In those days, the clinical use of the rays met with quite a few practical difficulties. One of them related to the dosage. James Ewing, whose book on neoplastic diseases remained a standard work ever since its first appearance in 1919 until after the Second World War, described the early history of radiation therapy in the following words. 'Much confusion arose from the multiplication of terms, the conflict of theories, and the striking differences in the effects of different doses. There was the stimulating dose, the erythema dose, the epilation dose, the vesicating dose and all too often the

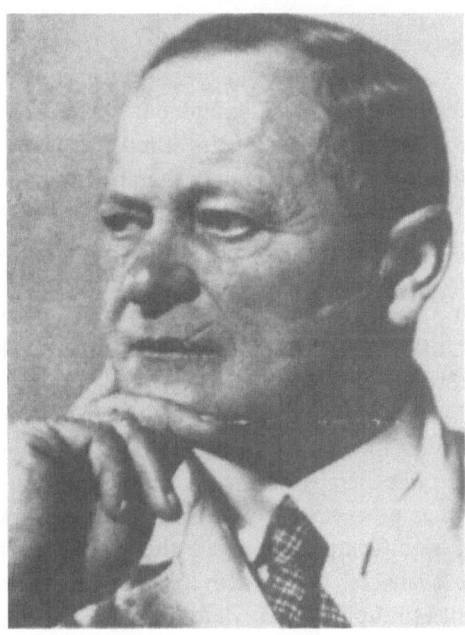

Fig. 37.   Hermann Gocht.

necrotizing dose'.[285] In spite of these difficulties, radiotherapy quickly became the treatment of choice in inoperable cases.

The introduction, in 1902, of a workable dosimeter by Guido Holzknecht (1872–1931) in Vienna, marked a great step forward. Holzknecht, who occupied himself in particular with the treatment of malignant diseases, died as a result of a roentgen lesion incurred at an early stage of his career. He was by no means the only one to die as a consequence of working with roentgen rays. In 1919, the first edition of the *Ehrenbuch der Röntgenologen und Radiologen aller Nationen* (the Book of Honour of Roentgenologists and Radiologists of all Nations) published by the journal *Strahlentherapie*, listed 169 physicians who paid with their lives for their all too close association with ionizing rays. In the second edition, which appeared in 1959, the list had expanded with another 190 names.[286]

The radiologist, as a medical specialist, first made his entrance in the eventful twenties. Before that, and in many cases even for many years afterwards, radiology was in the hands of clinicians. The word 'radiology' was coined in 1897 by the Frenchman Antoine Béclère (1852–1939) in Paris as a substitute for 'roentgenology', a somewhat uneasy word for non-German tongues. The Radiumhemmet (Radium-house) founded in Stockholm in 1910, and the Institut du Radium opened in Paris in 1914, indicated by their very names the importance attached to radiotherapy on the eve of the First World War. Many others were to follow.

Radiation was not for long reserved for inoperable cases of breast cancer. In the expectation that cancer cells that were left behind after the operation would be killed by rays, many hospitals in Europe and America started to use postoperative irradiation as an adjunct to surgery. In the light of our present techniques, the way this was done initially was quite inadequate, since the equipment which was in operation until the First World War had a voltage of 150 kilovolts at most. It was only after that war that apparatus better suitable for deep roentgen-ray therapy became available with voltages ranging from 170 to 200 kV. Radical mastectomy followed by X-ray became the standard treatment in numerous centres. Preoperative radiation for cases on the borderline of operability was introduced late in the twenties. In 1927, the Paris surgeon Robert Monod was surprised to find that an inoperable tumour which he had subjected to radiotherapy, afterwards lent itself well to surgery. The patient was in good condition more than three years afterwards.[287] Several authors, for instance Korteweg in 1916,[288] Perthes in 1920,[289] Harrington in 1929 – based on a follow-up of 1,859 cases treated at the Mayo Clinic from 1910 to 1923[290] – expressed their doubts on the value of additional radiotherapy. Their unsympathetic attitude towards ancillary radiation in operable cases proceeded from statistical returns which suggested that the use of X-ray had not significantly improved the overall results. Even after better apparatus had become available, the controversy remained, both the advocates and opponents using statistics to support their views.

Amongst the enthousiastic supporters of postoperative radiation were George Edward Pfahler (1874–1957) and his associate D.L. Parry in Philadelphia: in 1931 these authors advised its use in all cases starting two weeks after surgery.[291] But an analysis carried out by Pfahler three years later of 1,022 private cases treated from 1902 to 1928, demonstrated that, for patients belonging to Stage I, it made no significant difference whether they were treated by surgery combined with irradiation or by operation alone. In Stage II, however, the five-year survival of those who had the combined treatment was definitely better than that of the patients who underwent only surgery. Pfahler and others also stressed the importance of an accurate and careful radiation technique.[292] This emphasis had direct reference to fractionated irradiation, the most important advance in the practice of radiotherapy to be made – once again – in the eventful twenties following experimental work carried out in the Curie Foundation in Paris.

Although irradiation as the sole treatment of inoperable cases had been in almost general use ever since the early years of the century, in the 1920's few authors reported on their experiences in treating operable tumours by radiation only. In 1922, William Stephen Stone (1867–1946), an internist and radiumtherapist in the Memorial Hospital in New York City formally rejected radical surgery as a treatment of mammary cancer, since radiotherapy only would offer essentially better results, also in operable cases. He based this conclusion on his experiences with 10,000 cases of malignancy which had helped him to define the indications of radiotherapy.[293]

Fritz König (1866–1936), professor of surgery in Würzburg, combated such views by stating that the results of surgical treatment of Steinthal Stage I patients gave such a high percentage of radical cure, that it was not to be expected that radiotherapy as a sole treatment could ever do better. On the other hand, the outcome of ray treatment was superior in terms of prolonging life in Steinthal Stage III cases. Local recurrences might also benefit from irradiation. In Stage II, there were presumably patients who would be better off with X-ray only, but it was as yet impossible to distinguish between cases that would react favourably and those that would not.[294] König probably voiced the opinion of the majority of surgeons.

It is surprising that any radiotherapeutic cures were obtained at all in cases of breast cancer with the low-voltage X-ray machines available at the time. Significantly, Geoffrey Langdon Keynes (b. 1887) of St. Bartholomew's Hospital in London, used radium as a source of radiation. On the base of previous experiences gained with radium treatment as an adjunct to surgery, he extended its application to operable cases while leaving the scalpel in the cupboard. He claimed to have a five-year survival rate of 77.1 per cent in the absence of axillary nodes and of 36.3 per cent if the axilla was involved.[295]

In the 1930's super-voltage X-rays became available. The megaVolt apparatus introduced in 1939 in The Netherlands Cancer Institute, Antoni van Leeuwenhoekhuis in Amsterdam, for instance, was capable of generating roentgen-rays at a voltage of more than one million volts. This appliance – colloquially called 'the millionaire' – was for many years unique in Europe[296] (Fig. 38).

The introduction of super-voltage therapy led to the development of new methods of patient management with regard to the treatment of breast cancer, reflecting a growing reliance on the curative powers of the ionizing rays. This reliance was expressed in three different ways.

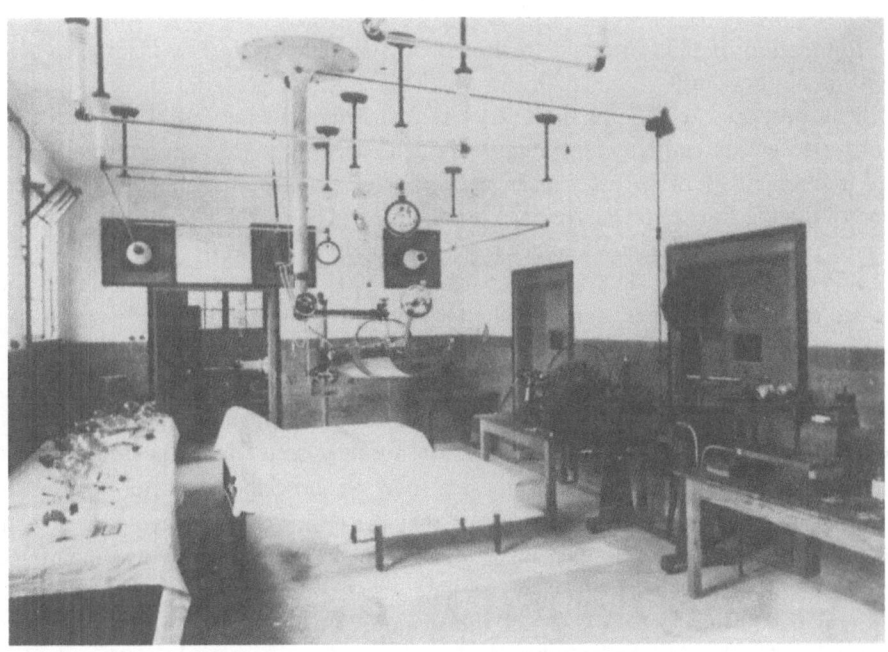

Fig. 38.   Philips megaVolt irradiation apparatus in The Netherlands Cancer Institute (1939).

Early champions of local excision of the tumour followed by adequate radiotherapy, were the French radiologist François Baclesse (1896–1967) and his co-workers. Between 1937 and 1953 they treated 100 Stage I and Stage II patients in this manner in the Fondation Curie in Paris. They concluded that the results were comparable to those of the orthodox treatment.[297]

A method somewhat comparable to the one just mentioned is simple mastectomy – ablatio simplex – followed by radical irradiation. Its proponent is Robert McWhirter (b. 1904), radiotherapist in Edinburgh. In TNM Stage I patients, he argued, radical mastectomy would overshoot the mark, whereas in Stage II, the same procedure might be inadequate since the disease often spreads beyond the axilla when the lymph nodes are involved.[298] The McWhirter technique gave rise to a flood of papers, both for and against, it seems to have its adherents especially in Great Britain.

A third approach, treatment by radiation alone, was adopted by Baclesse from 1936. In 1965 he reported his five-year results in 431 patients. For Columbia Stage A patients this amounted to 54 per cent survival, but for Columbia Stage B this rose to 61 per cent.[299]

After the development of higher voltage X-rays and the radio-active cobalt beam in the sixties, treatment by radiation preceded by local tumour excision – for which the ugly word 'lumpectomy' was invented – received much attention in America and in the European continent as well as elsewhere. This does not mean at all, however, that the traditional radical mastectomy with ancillary ray treatment has been relegated to the rubbish-heap of medicine.

Hormonal treatment

The foundation of the hormonal treatment of breast cancer too was laid even before the turn of the century. In 1889, Albert Schinzinger (1827–1911), in Freiburg im Breisgau, proposed to remove the ovaries in menstruant women prior to mastectomy in order to effect early ageing, because he had gained the experience from 96 cases that the prognosis of breast cancer is worse for younger patients.[300] This recommendation does not seem to have been observed.

A surgeon to the Glasgow Cancer Hospital, George Thomas Beatson (1848–1933), did, however, report in 1896 and once again in 1901 on the results of oophorectomy in cases of advanced breast cancer. When studying the phenomenon of lactation with a view to writing a M.D.-thesis, he found that the production of milk was not controlled by a special nerve-supply. He had learned that in some countries (Australia) it was the custom to remove the ovaries of the cows after calving in order to maintain the milk supply indefinitely. In Scotland, the farmers used to put the bull to the cow when the milk production was decreasing, two or three months after the calf was born, because they knew from experience that the ensuing pregnancy – during which the ovary is functionless, as Beatson realized – a copious milk flow was maintained. All this pointed, in Beatson's view, to one organ – the ovaries – controlling the secretion of another, separate organ, the mamma, in the absence of a distinct nerve connection. (It should be remembered, that the notion of internal secretion had just dawned; the term hormone did not exist as yet as it was only coined by Starling in

1905). When examining a lactating breast under a microscope, it struck his attention that its features were very much like those of cancer, with the exception that, during lactation, the proliferated epithelial cells would rapidly vacuolate, undergo fatty degeneration and form milk. In carcinoma the cells stopped short of that process, penetrated the walls of the ducts and invaded the surrounding tissue.

The difference in behaviour of the epithelial cells was apparently brought about by the absence of ovarian influence, in the case of lactation. Removal of the ovaries could therefore be expected to promote fatty degeneration of the cells and to stop their invasive tendency. Three cases of advanced breast cancer had responded favourably to oophorectomy. 'We must look in the female to the ovaries as the seat of the exciting cause of carcinoma, certainly of the mamma, in all probability of the female generative organs generally, and possibly of the rest of the body', Beatson concluded.[301] It is interesting to note, that he prescribed thyroid extract as an adjuvant. This drug was considered a powerful lymphatic stimulant. It would, he believed, affect the metabolism of the body cells, raising their tone and improving their vigour: this would lessen the chance of dissemination.[302]

Surgical castration was performed fairly frequently, in cases of advanced breast cancer in young women, by a number of surgeons during the first decade of the century, with varying success. One quarter to one third of the patients thus treated were said to have benefitted. After about 1914, interest in ovariectomy waned. This, according to MacMahon and Cahill, was due to radiation-castration, which had been introduced in 1905.[303] It may well have been that the unfavourable results of the latter procedure caused castration as such to fall into disrepute. At the same time that clinical ovariectomy receded to the background, the subject was taken up in the research laboratory. A brief summary of the most important work from the twenties and thirties is given on pages 91 to 94 in this book.

It can be said that the modern era of endocrine surgery started with the work of Huggins and his collaborators, when they reported the beneficial effects of castration on the growth of cancer of the prostrate (1940).[266] Huggins also reintroduced surgical oophorectomy to remove the main source of endogenous oestrogens.[304]

Since the adrenals appeared to be an additional source of steroid hormones which is not eliminated by removal of the gonads or by menopause, Huggins and his co-workers instituted bilateral adrenalectomy, once corticosteroids had become available for substitution, for cases of metastatic breast cancer that responded unfavourably to ovariectomy or were beyond menopause. Some, but by no means all of them responded by a striking remission. Also in the early fifties, Rolf Luft and Herbert Olivecrona (b. 1891) in Stockholm,[305] and shortly afterwards Olof H. Pearson and his associates at the Sloan-Kettering Institute in New York,[266] introduced hypophysectomy for advanced breast cancer: its benefits were comparable to those of adrenalectomy.

Non-operative hormonal treatment dates from 1939, when P. Ulrich described the beneficial effect produced by testosterone in two cases of breast cancer.[306] In 1944, Alexander John Haddow (b. 1912) and his collaborators in Edinburgh demonstrated the beneficial influence of synthetic oestrogen upon advanced malignant breast disease.[307]

The introduction of such compounds in clinical medicine had been preceded by some twenty years of intensive laboratory research, which in 1936 had finally resulted in the isolation of testosterone, the most important of the androgenic hormones, in the pharmacological laboratory of professor Ernst Laqueur (1880–1947) in Amsterdam, and its semi-synthesis shortly afterwards by other groups. In 1938 followed the discovery of stilboestrol, a substance with a biological action which is quite similar to that of oestrogenic hormones, by Edward Charles Dodds (1899–1973) in the Courtauld Institute, Middlesex Hospital. The structural formula of stilboestrol has received a place in heraldry, since it figures on the crest of Sir Edward Dodds' coat-of-arms, appearing in one of the stained glass windows in the magnificent Hall of the Society of Apothecaries in London.

Chemotherapy

As was shown in previous chapters, the use of chemical compounds, of arsenic in particular, in the treatment of breast cancer goes back to ancient times. Modern chemotherapy, however, is of recent date and started with the introduction of alkylating agents and antimetabolites in the sixties. In the beginning, when single chemotherapeutic agents were employed, the results were rather disappointing. Such drugs often had, moreover, undesirable side effects which reduced their palliative value. Ever since drugs of different type have been used in succession, chemotherapy appears to be a valuable adjuvant in the treatment of disseminated breast cancer.

Epilogue

It is not for the medical historian to give a description of the present state of affairs with regard to mammary cancer or to any other disease for that matter. Contemporary textbooks, monographs and articles, which are certainly not in short supply, will keep the interested reader abreast with the concepts and therapies of the day. For an excellent survey of the developments during the past decade, the reader is referred to a recent publication by Graig Henderson and George P. Cancellos.[308]

Before concluding, the present writer would like to recall a few of the typical aspects of breast cancer which presented themselves persistently all through the centuries, be it with varying emphasis, together with one or two historical elements which date from a more recent past. Some of these aspects result from the fact that the origin of the disease was — and, in fact, still is — largely unknown. In this regard the oncologist of today is more or less in the situation in which physicians were when they faced infectious diseases before the discovery of bacteria. All they could — and can — do is to collect as many empirical facts as possible by careful observation and try to fit them into a theoretical system which offers a satisfactory explanation of the data and which forms, at the same time, a basis for rational therapy.

One such theoretical system was humoral pathology which for many centuries satisfied even the best minds. The doctrine of the humours not only accounted for carcinogenesis, it also gave an elegant explanation of predisposition, of heredity, of the importance of a proper diet, of the influence of the patient's character and of sorrowful experiences. Even trauma could be fitted into this interplay of humours.

In a process of scientific development which took almost three centuries, humoral pathology was discarded and superseded by several other systems, and conceptions marked by key-words like irritability, natural philosophy, pathological anatomy, scientific materialism. The humours disappeared, but predisposition, heredity, dietary facts, character structure, sorrow and physical trauma remained as factors stimulating the disease. They only became a lot more difficult to explain. An attempt made by Rokitansky and others in the middle of the nineteenth century at re-introducing humoral conceptions by advancing blastema as a semifluid matrix from which cancer develops, was given short shrift by Virchow. With the rejection of cancer blastema, predisposition or diatheses lost their material basis as well. The conception as such lingers, however, although in the background and without a clear explanation.

Dietary influences on the origin of breast cancer are less emphasized than in the past, at least in scientific medicine today. The age-old belief that certain food items can promote cancer, whereas other dietary constituents are inhibitive lives on, however, in the public at large, as well as in alternative medicine. As long as the cause of cancer remains unknown, all sorts of theories, old and new, will be advanced and defended, by physicians as well as by the lay-public.

Thus it is interesting to note that physicians all through the ages are inclined to attribute to influences of the mind and of the character whatever they are unable to explain by somatic causes. Before the discovery of the tuberculosis bacillus, for instance, consumption was associated with a particular sensitive and passive personality. This applies also to cancer. In the 1930's, the Viennese psychoanalist Wilhelm Reich included cancer among the diseases 'resulting from the emotional plague in social life'. More recently, Olle Hagnell of the Department of Psychiatry of the University of Lund in Sweden, thought to have established a relationship between personality type and liability to cancer. Working with the dimensions of personality function, determined by the constitutional disposition of the central nervous system as elaborated by the late professor of psychiatry Henrik Sjöbring (1879–1956) in Lund, he found, in a prospective study of ten years, a much higher proportion of cancer cases in substable women than in the controls ($p < 0.05$). The substable group, having much in common with Kretschmer's cyclothymic type, consists of warm, hearty, social and industrious people, effectively engaged in everyday happenings.[309] The historian remembers that in the beginning of the nineteenth century, Alexis Boyer numbered sensibility and irritability of the central nervous system among his carcinogenic factors.

It has been pointed out in Chapter 8 that in the nineteenth century the belief prevailed, that consumption and cancer exclude each other. Tuberculosis was the great killer at the time. Cancer, although known and feared as a deadly disease all through the history of medicine, was quantitatively far less important. When towards the end of the century consumption started to decrease and life expectancy was increasing, cancer received more and more public attention. For the first time in history it was realized that society at large had to make a stand against cancer, just as it was doing against tuberculosis (Fig. 39). In the beginning of the twentieth century, important financial means and expensive specialized institutes were established to combat the disease.

In spite of the huge amounts of money spent on research and on treatment, in spite of untiring efforts by so many research workers and clinicians all over the world, in spite of the availability of advanced technical aids, the mortality of breast cancer has not been substantially reduced during the last thirty years.[310]

Breast cancer has long ceased to be a disease just between the patient and her doctor. Since the Second World War, the treatment of the disease has become more and more the responsibility of a medical team in which a number of disciplines are represented. Ever since, in the course of the eighteenth century, humoral pathology was superseded by the belief in a focal, localized genesis of cancer, early detection and treatment remained the basic philosophy. The introduction of mammography in the fifties ushered in an era of mass screening, the value of which, however, still remains to be seen.[311] So-called clinical trials are a modern attempt at letting numbers

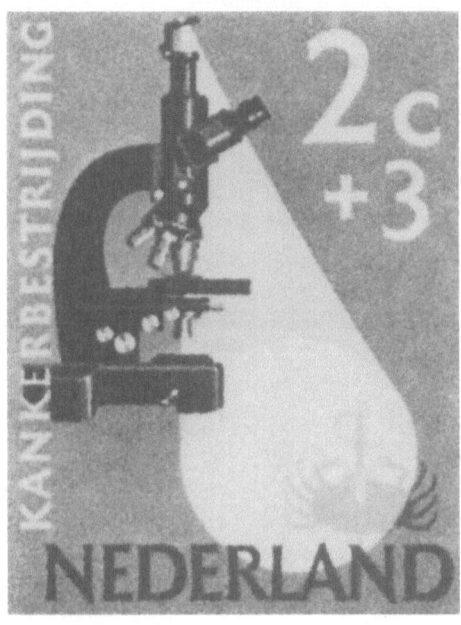

Fig. 39.   Dutch stamp issued in 1955 in aid of the anti-cancer campaign.

speak, since the returns of retrospective reviews appeared to be highly conflicting as to the best method of treatment.

The disappointing over-all results of the treatment of breast cancer in relation to the efforts and money invested since the beginning of the century, calls to mind one of Virchow's typical dictums: 'Es wird ja fleissig gearbeitet und viel mikroskopiert, aber es müsste mal wieder einer einen gescheiten Gedanken haben! (Indeed, a great deal of industrious work is being done and the microscope is extensively used, but someone should have another bright idea).[312] Perhaps somebody is nursing just such a bright idea right now.

Notes

1. Temkin O: The historiography of ideas in medicine. In: *Modern methods in the history of medicine.* Clark E (ed). London: Athlone Press University of London, 1971, p 1–21.
2. Wolff J: *Lehre von den Krebskrankheiten von den ältesten Zeiten bis zur Gegenwart.* 4 Teile in 5 Bde. Jena: G Fischer, 1907–1928.
3. Mansfield CM: *Early breast cancer.* Its history and results of treatment. Basel: S Karger, 1976.
4. Haagensen CD: *Diseases of the breast.* Philadelphia: WB Saunders, 1971².
5. Haagensen CD: An exhibit of important books, papers and memorabilia illustrating the evolution of the knowledge of cancer. *Am J Cancer* 18:42–126, 1933.
6. Hippocrates: Nature of man. In: *Hippocrates.* With an English translation by Jones WHS. 4 vols. Loeb Classical Library. Cambridge (Mass.): Harvard University Press; London: W Heinemann, 1953³, vol 4, p 11.
7. Hippocrates: Cinqième livre des épidémies, 101. In: *Oeuvres complètes d'Hippocrate.* Traduction nouvelle avec le texte grec en regard . . . par Littré E. 10 vols. Paris: J-B Baillière, 1839–1861, vol 5, p 258–259.
8. Hippocrates: Des maladies des femmes, II, 133. In: Littré (ed), vol 8, p 282–283.
9. Hippocrates: Aphorisms, VI, 38. In: Jones (ed), vol 4, p 189.
10. Michler M: *Die alexandrinischen Chirurgen.* Wiesbaden: F Steiner, 1968, p 7, 12.
11. Michler: *Op. cit.,* p 9.
12. Michler: *Op. cit.,* p 36–37.
13. Celsus: De medicina, V, 28. In: *Celsus de medicina.* With an English translation by Spencer WG. 3 vols. Loeb Classical Library. London: W Heinemann; Cambridge (Mass.): Harvard University Press, 1953², vol 2, p 129.
14. Aetius: *Aetii medici graeci contractae ex veteribus medicinae tetrabiblos. . . id est, sermones sedecim, per Janum Cornarium. . . conscripti,* IV, 43, 50. Lugduni: Ex officina. . . Beringorum fratrum, 1549, column 980, 983.
15. Aetius: Cancrorum curatio citra chirurgiam. *Op. cit.,* IV, 47, column 982.
16. Haddow A: Historical notes on cancer from the MSS of Louis Westenra Sambon. *Proc roy Soc Med* 29, 1015–1028, 1936.
17. Aetius: Cancri chirurgia, Leonidae; and: Cancri curatio post amputationem & inustionem. *Op. cit.,* IV, 45, 46, column 981.
18. Galen: De tumoribus praeter naturam, 12–14. In: *Opera omnia,* editionem curavit Kühn CG (Greek text with Latin translation by Chartier R). 20 vols in 22. Lipsiae: C Knobloch, 1821–1833, vol 7, p 726–728.
19. Galen: In Hippocratis librum de alimento commentarius, III, 17. In: Kühn (ed), vol 15, p 330.
20. Galen: Definitiones medicae (pseudo-Galenic) nr 385, 393. In: Kühn (ed), vol 19, p 442, 443.
21. Galen: *Op. cit.* (19), p 330.
22. Galen: Ad Glauconem de medendi methodo, II, 12. In: Kühn (ed), vol 11, p 139–144.
23. Galen: *Op. cit.* (19), p 327.
24. Galen: *Op. cit.* (19), p 327 and *op. cit.* (22), p 139.

25. Galen: *Op. cit.* (22), p 141.

26. Paul of Aegina: *The seven books of Paulus Aeginata.* Translation with a commentary... by Adams F. 3 vols. London: The Sydenham Society, 1844, vol 1, p 609–614.

27. Galen: *Op. cit.* (22), p 143.

28. Galen: *Op. cit.* (22), p 143 and *op. cit.* (19), p 88.

29. Galen: In Hippocratis aphorismos commentarius, 38. In: Kühn (ed), vol 28/1, p 59–61.

30. Galen: De methodo medendi, XIV, 9. In: Kühn (ed), vol 10, p 979.

31. Schonack W: *Die Rezepte des Scribonius Largus.* Jena: G Fischer. 1913.

32. Ovid: *Metamorphoses*, II, verse 825–832.

33. Pirenne H: *Histoire économique et sociale du Moyen-Age.* Paris: Presses Universitaires de France, 1969², p 1–12.

34. Codex Augiensis CXX, fol 98r–102r. Badische Landesbibliothek, Karlsruhe. Edited and translated by De Moulin D. In: *De heelkunde in de vroege Middeleeuwen* (Surgery in the early Middle Ages). Leiden: EJ Brill, 1964, p 52–79.

35. Gregoire de Nysse: *Vie de Sainte Macrime,* 31. Introduction, texte critique, traduction par Marval P. Sources chrétiennes 178. Les Editions du Cerf, 1971, p 243–247.

36. Augustine St: *De civitate Dei,* XXII, 8, 3.

37. Deubner L: *Kosmas und Damian.* Texte und Einleitung. Leipzig: 1907. Quoted by Heinemann K: Die Ärzteheiligen Kosmas und Damian. Ihre Wunderheilungen im Lichte alter und neuer Medizin. *Med-hist J* 9, 255–317, 1974.

38. Abulcasis: *La chirurgie d'Abulcasis,* II, 53. Traduite par Leclerq L, Paris: 1861. Quoted by Gurlt E: *Geschichte der Chirurgie.* 3 vols. Berlin: A Hirschwald, 1898, vol 1, p 631.

39. Guglielmo da Saliceto: *Chirurgia,* I, 58. Italian translation by Tabanelli M in: *La chirurgia italiana nell' alto medioevo.* 2 vols. Firenze: LS Olschki, 1965, vol 2, p 609–611.

40. Bruno da Longoburgo: *Chirurgia magna,* I, 16. Cited by Gurlt: *Op. cit.* (38), vol 1, p 730.

41. Teodorico Borgognoni: *The surgery of Theodoric,* III, 7. Translation from the Latin by Campbell E and Colton J. 2 vols. New York: Appleton Century Crofts, 1955–1960, vol 2, p 31.

42. Henri de Mondeville: *Chirurgie de Maître Henri de Mondeville,* I, 7. Traduction française par Nicaise E. Paris: F Alcan. 1893, p 57.

43. Henri de Mondeville: *Op. cit.,* II, 4, p 468–481; 8, p 704–708.

44. Paré A: *De chirurgie ende alle de opera,* VII, 26–33. (Dutch translation by Battus C of the *Oeuvres complètes.* 1575). Dordrecht: J Canin, 1592, p 264–273.

45. Paré: *Op. cit.,* p 269.

46. Haddow: *Op. cit.* (16), p 1025. Communicated by Dr. Cornelius Bonne, then pathologist at the Netherlands Cancer Institute in Amsterdam.

47. Paré: *Op. cit.,* p 271.

48. Fabricius Hildanus: *Observationum et curationum chirurgicarum centuriae, Cent* II. Lugduni: IA Huguetan, 1641, p 267–269.

49. Scultetus J: *Armamentarium chirurgicum,* Tab 38. Venetiis: Combi & La Nou, 1665, p 137.

50. Arceo, F: *De recta curandorum vulnerum ratione,* II, 3. Antverpiae: 1574. Quoted by Gurlt: *Op. cit.* (38), III, p 387.

51. Falloppio G: *Opera genuina omnia.* 3 vols in 1. Venetiis: Apud Jo Antonium & Jacobum de Franciscis, 1606².
Falloppio's views on malignancy were clearly exposed by Rather JL, in his *The genesis of cancer.* Baltimore and London: The Johns Hopkins University Press. 1978, p 14–19. Rather used the first edition of the collected works (Frankfurt: 1600).

52. Falloppio: *Op. cit.,* vol 3, p 79r–81v.

53. Falloppio: *Op. cit.,* vol 2, p 67r–77r.

54. Falloppio: *Op. cit.,* vol 3, p 90v–92r.

55. Rothschuh KE: *Konzepte der Medizin in Vergangenheit und Gegenwart.* Stuttgart: Hippokrates Verlag, 1978, p 224–228.

56. Rather: *Op. cit.* (51), p 31.

110

57. De Le Boë Sylvius F: *Opera medica*. Amsterdam: D Elsevirius & Abr Wolfgang, 1680², p 158–390.
   An excellent survey of Sylvius' physiology and pathophysiology is given by King LS in: *The road to medical enlightenment*. London: MacDonald; New York: American Elsevier, 1970, p 93–136.
58. Rothschuh: *Op. cit.* (55), p 235.
59. De Le Boë Sylvius: *Op. cit.* (57), Appendix Tract III: De lue venera, p 667.
60. Hoffmann F: *Fundamenta medicinae ex principiis naturae mechanicis in usum philiatrorum succinte proposita*, II, 6. Halle: SJ Hübner, 1695. Quoted by King: *Op. cit.* (57), p 199.
61. Dionis P: *Verhandeling van alle de chirurgicale operatien, na de nieuwste, zekerste, en gemakkelijkste manier*. (Dutch translation of *Cours d'opérations de chirurgie, demonstrées au Jardin Royal*. Paris: 1707). Rotterdam: Joannes Hofhout, 1710.
62. Alliot JB: *Traité du cancer, sa nature et les moyens pour le guérir méthodiquement*. Paris: 1698. Quoted by Dionis: *Op. cit.*, p 347–348.
63. Gendron CD: *Recherches sur la nature et la guérison des cancers*. Paris: 1700. Quoted by Dionis: *Op. cit.* (61), p 345.
   It should be noted that the feeling that cancer is a 'cold disease' persists even today in alternative medicine.
64. Helvetius A: *Traité des pertes de sang avec leur remède spécifique et une lettre sur la guérison du cancer*. Paris: 1697. Quoted by Dionis: *Op. cit.* (61), p 346 and 348–349.
65. Devaux J: *Suplément et suite d l'Index funereus chirurgicorum*. Ms 2190 Bibl interuniv de médecine. Paris. p 478.
66. Dionis: *Op. cit.* (61), p 353.
67. Tulp N: *Observationes medicae*, IV, 8. Amsterdam: 1652. (A fifth edition used by us appeared in Leyden (J du Vivie) as late as 1716, p 292–294).
68. Bandaline J: *La lutte internationale contre le cancer*. Paris: N Maloine, 1933, p 50.
69. Bierens de Haan JCJ: Mondelinge mededeling aan I de Bruijn. In: *Catalogus van de verzameling etsen van Rembrandt in het bezit van I de Bruijn en JG de Bruijn-van der Leeuw*. De Bruijn I. 's Gravenhage: Martinus Nijhoff, 1932, p 187.
70. Haneveld GT: *Mr Arnoldus Fey, chirurgijn tot Oirschot*. Amsterdam: Meesters, 1977, p 41.
71. Körbler J: *Geschichte der Krebskrankheit*. Wien: H Ranner, 1973, p 40–42.
72. Ward J: *Diary of the Rev John Ward, A.M., vicar of Stratford-upon-Avon, extending from 1648 to 1679*. From the original MSS preserved in the Library of The Medical Society in London. Arranged by Severn Ch. London: H Colburn, 1839, p 244–247.
73. De Moulin D, de Groot IM: The cancer operation by Romeyn de Hooghe. *Organorama* 5 (11), 22–23, 1974.
74. Van Horne J: *Microtechne id est brevissima chirurgiae methodus*. Lugd Batav. 1663, p 91.
75. Bidloo G: *Opera omnia*. Lugd Batav: S Luchtmans, 1715, p 1–216.
76. Heister L: *Heelkundige onderwijzingen*. (Dutch translation from the German: *Chirurgie*. Nuremberg. 1718, with notes and comments by Ulhoorn H). 2 vols. Amsterdam: Janssoons van Waesbergen, 1714, vol 3, p 845–856.
77. Morgagni JB: *De sedibus et causis morborum per anatomen indagatis libri quinque*. 4 vols. Lovani: Typographia Academica, 1767, vol 4, p 31, 41–46.
78. Wiseman R: *Eight surgical treatises*. 2 vols. London: B Motte, 1734⁶, vol 1, p 164–195.
79. Gahrliep GC: De carcinomate latente, deliberato consilio, sed infausto sidere, dextera satis manu, dubio diu successu, funesto tandem exitu extirpato. *Ephemerides naturae curiosorum dec III*, 5/6:370–374, 1698.
80. Le Cat CN: Mémoire sur la question proposée par l'Académie royale de Chirurgie pour le prix de 1739, si l'on doit amputer le carcinôme des mammelles. In: *Recueil des pièces qui ont concouru pour le prix de l'Académie royale de Chirurgie*. Paris: Delaguette, 1753, vol 1, p 241–267.
81. Hevin P: *Cours de pathologie et de thérapeutique chirurgicales*. Paris: Méquignon, 1785, p 312–324.

82. De Moulin D: On the early history of antisepsis. *Arch Chir Neerl* 31:197–201, 1979.
83. Boerhaave H: *Praelectiones academicae in proprias institutiones rei medicae*. Edidit et notas addidit Haller A. 6 vols. Gottingae: A Vandenhoeck, 1794, vol 6, p 278–279.
84. Astruc J: *Traité des maladies des femmes*. 6 vols. Paris: PG Cavelier, 1770², vol 5, p 314–339.
85. Hoffmann F: *Medicinae rationalis systematicae tomi quarti . . .* 4 vols. Francoforti ad Moenum: F Varrentrapp, 1739, vol 4, p 249–289.
86. Goethe JW: *Wilhelm Meisters Lehrjahre*, V, 16. 1795/1796.
87. King LS: *The medical world of the eighteenth century*. Huntington NY: RE Krieger, 1971², p 59–121.
88. De Gorter J: *De gezuiverde heelkonst*, VII, 2. Leiden: De Janssoons van der Aa, 1735, p 393.
89. Van Swieten GLB: *Verklaaring der korte stellingen van Herman Boerhaave*. 2 vols. (Dutch translation of *Commentaria in Hermanni Boerhaave Aphorismos. . .* (Lugd Batav. 1742–1776). Leiden: J & H Verbeek, 1768, vol 1 (2), p 586–642).
90. De Gorter: *Op. cit.* (88), p 125.
91. Rather: *Op. cit.* (51), p 13.
92. Boerhaave H: *Kortbondige spreuken wegens de ziektens*, Aphor 392. (Dutch translation from the Latin *Aphorismi de cognoscendis et curandis morbis*. Lugd Batav. 1709) Amsterdam: Joh Gysius, 1741, p 67. Reprint 'Librye der Geneeskunst' I. Alphen a/d Rijn: Stafleu, 1979.
93. Dobson J: John Hunter's views on cancer. *Ann R Coll Surg Engl* 1:176–181, 1959.
94. Van Swieten: *Op. cit.* (89), p 597.
95. Le Dran HF: Du cancer des mammelles. In: *Encyclopédie ou dictionnaire universel raisonné des connoisances humaines*, mis en ordre par [FB] Félice. 57 vols. Yverdon: 1770–1780, vol 27, p 314–316. This is a Protestant pirate edition of Diderot's and d'Alembert's famous encyclopaedia.
96. Quesnay F: Mémoire sur les vices des humeurs. *Mèm Acad roy Chir* 1:1–154, 1743.
97. Le Dran HF: Mémoire avec un précis de plusieurs observations sur le cancer. *Mèm Acad roy Chir* 3:1–54, 1757.
98. Schrage AS: Bekroond antwoord op de vraag: 'kunnen wij ons overtuigd houden, dat een waare kanker immer zonder de afsetting tot genezing is gebracht?' (Prize-winning answer to the question: 'can we be certain that a true cancer was ever cured without amputation?'). *Hand Geneesk Genootsch 'Servandis Civibus'* 4:207–286, 1779.
99. Guy R: *Practical observations on cancers and disorders of the breast*. London: 1762. Quoted by Wolff: *Op. cit.* (2), vol 1, p 67.
100. Astruc: Quoted by Wolff: *Op. cit.* (2), vol 1, p 63.
101. De Gorter: *Op. cit.* (88), p 400.
102. Heister: *Op. cit.* (76), p 378–387.
103. Louis A: Observations & remarques sur les effets du virus carcinomateux. *Mèm Acad roy Chir* 3:88–91, 1757.
104. Van den Block [?]: Waarnemingen omtrent het inwendig gebruik der onlangs aangeprezen middelen tot genezing van de kanker in 't borst (Observations on the internal use of remedies that were of late recommended for curing the cancer of the breast). *Uitgezochte Verhand Societeiten Wetensch* 6:315–329, 1761.
105. Le Dran HF: Cancer. In: *Encyclopédie* (95), vol 7, p 229–235.
106. Peyrilhe B: *Dissertatio academica de cancro*. Parisiis: De Hansy Jeune, 1774.
107. Grashuys J: *Exercitatio medico-chirurgica de scirrho et carcinomate*. Amstelaedami: I Tirion, 1741.
108. Van Gesscher D: *Proeve over de voornaamste langdurige gezwellen*. Amsterdam: J. Morterre, 1767, p 22–34.
109. Petit JL: *Oeuvres posthumes de chirurgie*, mises au jour par M Lesne [FD]. 3 vols. Paris: Prault, 1774², vol 1, p 230.
110. Camper P: Over den waren aart der kankervorming en over een zeer zakelijk en onfeilbaar teken van onherstelbaaren borstkanker (On the true nature of carcinogenesis and on a very pertinent and infallible sign of incurable breast cancer). *Genees-, Nat-, Huishoudk Kabinet* 2:193–208, 1779.

111. De Gorter: *Op. cit.* (88), p 401.

112. Heister: *Op. cit.* (76), vol 1, p 371–378.

113. De Lassone JMF: An instituenda cancri mammarum sectio? In: *Recueil des pièces qui ont concouru pour le prix de l'Académie royale de Chirurgie*. Paris: Delaguette, vol 1, p 269–295.

114. De Gorter: *Op. cit.* (88), p 402.

115. Petit JL: *Heelkundige grondbeginselen* (Fundamentals of surgery. Dutch translation by Morand P). Amsterdam: G Bom, 1772, p 132–136.

116. Hewson W: *Experimental enquiries:* Part the second. Containing a description of the lymphatic system in the human subject and other animals. London: J. Johnson, 1774.

117. Mascagni P: *Vasorum lymphaticorum corporis humani historia et ichnographia*. Senis: Ex typ P Carli, 1787.

118. *Encyclopédie:* cf (95).

119. Van Swieten: *Op. cit.* (89), p 643–707.

120. Van Wij GJ: Bekroond antwoord op prijsvraag: 'Kunnen wij ons overtuigd houden, dat een waare kanker immer zonder de afzetting tot genezing is gebracht?' (Prize-winning essay on: 'Can we be certain that a true cancer has ever been cured without amputation?') *Hand Geneesk Genootsch 'Servandis Civibus'* 4:3–206, 1779.

121. Pope A: On Mrs Corbet. In: *Collected Poems*. Edited by Bonamy Dobrée. Everyman's Library 760. London: JM Dent & Sons; New York: EP Dutton & Co, 1956², p 120.

122. Van Swieten: *Op. cit.* (89), p 643–707.

123. Hevin: *Op. cit.* (81), p 295–320.

124. De Gorter: *Op. cit.* (88), p 406.

125. Astruc: *Op. cit.* (84), vol 5, p 340–368.

126. Richter: Quoted by Fischer G: *Chirurgie vor 100 Jahren*. Leipzig: FCW Vogel, 1876, p 467. Reprint Berlin: Springer Verlag, 1978.

127. Brisbane J: *Select cases in the practice of medicine*. London: T Cadell, 1773, p 35.
Duncan A: *Medical cases*. Edinburgh: 1778, p 105. Quoted by Wolff: *Op. cit.* (2), vol 3/II, p 299.

128. Fischer CAF: Die Drüsenübel im weiblichen Busen. *J. Chir Augenheilk* 5:576–602, 1823.

129. Von Störck A: *Libellus quo demonstratur cicutam non solum usu interno tutissime exhiberi, sed et esse simul remedium valde utile in multis morbis qui hucusque curatu impossibiles dicebantur*. Vindebonae: JT Trattner, 1760.

130. Lambergen T: *Lectio inauguralis sistens ephemeridem persanati carcinomatis*. Groningae: Apud Henricum Vechnerum, 1754.

131. Dionis: *Op. cit.* (61), p 353.

132. Hunter: Quoted by Dobson: *Op. cit.* (93), p 179.

133. Richter: Quoted by Fischer: *Op. cit.* (126), p 466.

134. Hunter: Quoted by Dobson: *Op. cit.* (93), p 180.

135. Fearon: Quoted by Dobson: *Op. cit.* (93), p 181.

136. Bell B: *A system of surgery*. 6 vols. Edinburgh: Bell, Bradfute; London: GGJ & J Robinson, J Murray. 1791⁵, vol 5, p 436–460.

137. Petit: *Op. cit.* (109), vol 1, p 223–239.

138. De Montesquieu CL: *Oeuvres complètes*. 3 vols. Masson A (ed). Paris: Nagel, 1955, vol 3, p 1401.

139. Prov Bibl Zeeland (Middelburg). MS 6262, supplementary sheet. 1772 (?).

140. Van der Haar J: *Verhandeling over de natuur en aart van de klier-, knoest-, en kankergezwellen* (Treatise on the nature of glandular, scirrhous and cancerous tumours). Amsterdam: J Heun, 1761.

141. Doets CJ: *De heelkunde van Petrus Camper 1722–1789*. Thesis Leiden: 1948, p 25.

142. Monro A: Collections of blood in cancerous breasts. In: *The works of Alexander Monro*. Published by his son Alexander Monro. Edinburgh: Ch Elliot, 1781, p 484–491.

143. Hill: Quoted by Wolff: *Op. cit.* (2), vol 4, p 20.
It seems somewhat doubtful though whether Hill really referred to breast cancer only, as Wolff wrote. I have not been able to consult Hill's *Cases in surgery*. Edinburgh: 1772, but

Boyer, writing in 1818, stated that only five of Hill's cases referred to cancer of the breast. Of these, only two were apparently cured. Boyer's contributions are discussed on p 53 and 54.

144. Richter: Cited by Fischer: *Op. cit.* (126), p 464.

145. Bandaline: *Op. cit.* (68), p 305–318.

146. Haubold H: Alte Zeitungsberichte über den Krebs. *Monatschr Krebsbekämpfung* 8:15–17, 1940.

147. Gelfand T: *The training of surgeons in eighteenth-century Paris and its influence on medical education.* Ann Arbor (Mich): Univ Microfilms International, 1979, p 278.

148. Ackerknecht EH: Pariser Chirurgie von 1794 bis 1850. *Gesnerus* 17:137–144, 1960.

149. Crosse VM: *A surgeon in the early nineteenth century.* Edinburgh and London: E & S Livingstone, 1868, p 33, 39.

150. Brown J: *Rab and his friends.* New York: H.M. Caldwell, nd. For the greater part reprinted in: *Sourcebook of medical history.* Clendening L. New York: Dover Publ., 1960, p 346–354.

151. Forster EM: *Marianne Thornton.* A domestic biography. London: E. Arnold, 1956, p 134.

152. Boyer A: *Traité des maladies chirurgicales et des opérations qui leur conviennent.* 11 vols. Paris: Migneret, 1818–1826.

153. Boyer: *Op. cit.,* vol 2, p 354.

154 Boyer: *Op. cit.,* vol 2, p 341.

155. Ackerknecht EH: Diathesis: the word and the concept in medical history. *Bull Hist Med* 56:317–325, 1982.

156. Boyer: *Op. cit.,* vol 7, p 223.

157. Boyer: *Op. cit.,* vol 2, p 357

158. Boyer: *Op. cit.,* vol 7, p 237–239.

159. Roux PJ: Mémoire renfermant quelques vues générales sur le cancer. In: *Oeuvres chirurgicales de PJ Desault.* Bichat X. 3 vols. Paris: Méquignon, 1803², vol 3, p 406–439.

160. Bayle CL, Cayol JB: Cancer. In: *Dictionnaire des sciences médicales.* 12 vols. Paris: Craput & Panckoucke, 1812–1822, vol 3, p 537–679.

161. Crosse: *Op. cit.* (149), p 80.

162. Logger HJ: Aanteekeningen op eene wetenschappelijke reize naar Parijs, in den jare 1818 (Notes on a scientific journey to Paris, made in 1818) *Geneesk Bijdr* 1:96–146, 1826.

163. Hemlow J: *The journal and letters of Fanny Burney.* 10 vols. London: Oxford Univ Press, 1972-, vol 5, p 596–615. Mrs Burney's case was discussed by Moore AR: Preanesthetic mastectomy: a patient's experience. *Surgery* 83:200–205, 1978.

164. Haneveld GT: Compression as a treatment of cancer, a historical survey. *Arch chir neerl* 31:1–8, 1979.

165. Bichat X: *Anatomie générale, appliquée à la physiologie et la médecine.* 2 vols. Paris: Ladrange, Lheureux, 1818², vol 2, p 134.

166. Beclard PF: Tissus accidentels. In: *Anatomie générale etc.* Bichat X. Nouvelle édition par Béclard et augmentée d'un grand nombre de notes nouvelles par F Blandin. 4 vols. Paris: JS Chaude, 1830, vol 4, p 539–546.

167. Laennec RTH: Anatomie pathologique. In: *Dictionnaire des sciences médicales.* Referred to under nr 160. Vol 2.
Quoted by Wolff: *Op. cit.* (2), vol 1, p 92–94. For a more thorough discussion of Laennec's views on tumours see Rather: *Op. cit.* (51), p 60–64.

168. Cruveilhier J: *Essai sur l'anatomie pathologique en général.* Paris: 1816 and: Description anatomique de cancers. *Bull Soc Anat Paris* 1827 (cancer juice). Quoted by Wolff: *Op. cit.* (2), vol 1, p 107–109.

169. Rooseboom M: Microscopium. Leiden: Rijksmuseum voor de Geschiedenis der Natuurwetenschappen, 1956.

170. Müller J: *Über den feinern Bau und die Formen der krankhaften Geschwülste.* Lief 1. Berlin: G. Reimer, 1838.

171. Hannover A: Bericht über die Leistungen in der skandinavischen Literatur im Gebiete der Anatomie und Physiologie in den Jahren 1841–1843. *Arch Anat Phys wiss Med* 11:1–49, 1844, p 18–20.

172. Lebert H: *Physiologie pathologique.* 2 vols. Paris: JB Baillière, 1845, vol 2, p 254–260.
173. Lebert H: *Traité pratique des maladies cancéreuses et des affections curables confondues avec le cancer.* Paris: JB Baillière, 1851. Review by S [chrant JM] in: *Ned Weekbl Geneesk* 1:446–447, 1851.
174. Velpeau AALM: *Traité des maladies du sein et de la région mammaire.* Paris: V Masson, 1854.
175. Velpeau: *Op. cit.,* p 421.
176. Hey W: *Practical observations in surgery.* London: 1814³. Quoted by Wolff: *Op. cit.* (2), p 84–85.
177. Velpeau: *Op. cit.,* p 448.
178. Velpeau: *Op. cit.,* p 454.
179. Velpeau: *Op. cit.,* p 481–504.
180. Velpeau: *Op. cit.,* p 491.
181. Velpeau: *Op. cit.,* p 578.
182. Schrant JM: Het vraagstuk van den kanker voor de Académie de Médecine te Parijs (The problem of cancer in the Académie de Médecine in Paris). *Ned Weekbl Geneesk* 5:141–145, 1855.
    Schrant's extensive report – there were several instalments – was based on a series of articles in the *Gazette médicale de Paris.*
183. Vogel J: Pathologische Anatomie des menschlichen Körpers. I Abtheil, vol 8, p 258. In: *Vom Baue des menschlichen Körpers.* Bischoff WTh, Henle J, Huschke E, Theile FW, Valentin G, Vogel J, Wagner R (eds). Leipzig: L Voss, 1845.
184. Rokitansky C: *Handbuch der pathologischen Anatomie.* 3 vols; Wien: Braumüller & Seidler, 1842–1846, vol 1 (1846), p 552–556.
185. Paget J: *Lectures on surgical pathology,* revised and edited by Turner W. London: Longman Green Longman Roberts & Green, 1863, p 766.
186. Virchow R: *Die Cellularpathologie in ihrer Begründung auf physiologische und pathologische Gewebelehre.* Berlin: A Hirschwald, 1858.
187. Remak R: Über extracelluläre Entstehung thierischer Zellen und über die Vermehrung derselben durch Theilung. *Arch Anat Physiol wiss Med* 28:47–57, 1852.
188. Virchow R: *Die krankhaften Geschwülste.* 3 vols. Berlin: A Hirschwald, 1863–1873, Vol 1, p 26–27.
189. Virchow: *Op. cit.,* p 28.
190. Virchow: *Op. cit.,* p 92.
191. Virchow: *Op. cit.,* p 35.
192. Remak: Quoted by Wolff: *Op. cit.* (2), vol 1, p 221.
193. Thiersch C: *Der Epithelialkrebs namentlich der Haut.* Leipzig: W Engelmann, 1865.
194. Waldeyer-Hartz HWG: Die Entwicklung der Carcinome. *Virchows Arch path Anat* 41:470–523, 1867; 55:67–159, 1872.
195. Dietrich A: Marksteine der Krebsforschung. *Klin Wschr* 15:1297–1300, 1936.
196. Tillmanns H: Die Ätiologie und Histogenese des Carcinoms. [Langenbecks] *Arch klin Chir* 50:507–534, 1895.
197. Tillmanns: *Op. cit.,* p 510–513.
198. Hansemann: Cited by Wolff: *Op. cit.* (2), vol 1, p 470–471.
199. Speculations on a possible parasitic origin already existed in the seventeenth century, as we read in Dionis: *Op. cit.* (61), p 343, and were revived by Joseph Adams (1756–1817) in London in his *Observations on the cancerous breast* (London: 1801, quoted by Virchow: *Op. cit.* (188), p 18), but exercised in their time but little influence. Interestingly, Adams was inspired by work of John Hunter on hydatid disease.
200. Jensen CO: Experimentelle Untersuchungen über Krebs bei Mäusen (Danish). *Hospitals-tidende.* 1903, p 549–581. Abstracted by Scheel V in: *Centralbl allg Path path Anat* 14:815, 1903.
201. Onuigbo WIB: A history of the cell theory of cancer metastasia. *Gesnerus* 20:90–95, 1963.
202. Wilder RJ: The historical development in the concept of metastasis. *J M. Sinai Hosp* 23:728–734, 1956.

203. Paget J: In: Discussion on cancer. *Transact path Soc London* 25:287−402, 1874, p 314−328.
204. Wolff: *Op. cit.* (2), vol 1, p 359.
205. Billroth Th: *Die Krankheiten der Brustdrüsen.* Stuttgart: F Enke, 1880.
206. Billroth: *Op. cit.*, p 95−96.
207. Billroth: *Op. cit.*, p 98.
208. Billroth: *Op. cit.*, p 116−117.
209. Duvillard EE: *Analyse et tableaux de l'influence de la petite vérole sur la mortalité à chaque âge, et de celle qu'un préservatif tel que la vaccine peut avoir sur la population et la longevité.* Paris: Imprimerie Impériale, 1806.
210. Louis PCA: *Recherches sur les effets de la saignée dans quelques maladies inflammatoires, et sur l'action de l'émétique et des vésicatoires dans la pneumonie.* Paris: JB Baillière, 1835.
211. Scotto J and Bailar III JC: Rigoni-Stern and medical statistics. A nineteenth-century approach to cancer research. *J Hist Med all Sci* 24:65−75, 1969.
212. Von Winiwarter A: *Beiträge zur Statistik der Carcinome* mit besonderer Rücksicht auf die dauerende Heilbarkeit durch operative Behandlung. Stuttgart: F Enke, 1878.
213. Billroth: *Op. cit.* (205), p 115−116.
214. Billroth: *Op. cit.*, p 135.
215. Billroth: *Op. cit.*, p 138.
216. Rokitansky: *Op. cit.* (184), vol 1, p 424−425.
217. Churchill JF: *A letter to the Registrar-General on the increase of cancer in England and its cause.* London: D. Stott, 1888.
218. Fischer: *Op. cit.* (128).
219. Virchow: *Op. cit.* (188), p 82.
220. Vanden Corput BE: Considérations sur l'étiologie du cancer et sur sa prophylaxie. *Bull Acad roy Belg* 11:1143−1175, 1883.
221. *Tableaux statistiques concernant la mortalité par cancer à Amsterdam,* pendant les périodes 1862−1867, 1872−1877, 1886−1890 et 1897−1902. Amsterdam: 1908.
222. Dieffenbach JF: *De operatieve chirurgie.* 2 vols. Utrecht: Kemink & Zn, 1846−1850 (Dutch translation of *Die operative Chirurgie.* Leipzig: 1844−1847), vol 2, p 371.
223. Schrant: *Op. cit.* (182), p 111−115.
224. Velpeau: *Op. cit.* (174), p 591.
225. Leroy d'Etiolles JJJ: Une lettre de M. Leroy d'Etiolles sur l'extirpation des tumeurs cancéreuses. *Bull Acad Méd* 9:454−458, 1844.
226. Statistiek van den kanker (Cancer statistics). *Ned Weekl Geneesk* 2:275 and 410, 1852.
227. Moore CH: On the influence of inadequate operations on the theory of cancer. *Med-chir Transact* 50:245−280, 1867.
228. Pancoast J: *A treatise on operative surgery.* Philadelphia: Carcy & Hart, 1844. Quoted by d'Arcy Power: *Op. cit.* (238), p 40.
229. Volkmann R: *Beiträge zur Chirurgie,* anschliessend an einen Bericht über die Thätigkeit der chirurgischen Universitäts-Klinik zu Halle im Jahre 1873. Leipzig: Breitkopff & Härtel, 1875, p 320−332.
230. Billroth: *Op. cit.* (205), p 151−153.
231. Billroth: *Op. cit.* (205), p 155.
232. Gross SW: An analysis of two hundred and seven cases of carcinoms of the breast. *Med News Philad* 51:613−616, 1887.
233. Heidenhain L: Ueber die Ursachen der localen Krebsrecidive nach Amputatio Mammae. [Langenbeck's] *Arch Klin Chir* 39:97−166, 1889.
234. Haagensen: *Op. cit.* (4), p 48.
235. Heidenhain: *Op. cit.* (233), p 155−156.
236. Halsted WS: The results of operations for the cure of cancer of the breast performed at The Johns Hopkins Hospital from June, 1889 to January, 1894. *Johns Hopkins Hosp Rep* 4:297−350, 1894−1895.
237. Meyer W: An improved method of the radical operation for carcinoma of the breast. *Med Rec* 46:746−749, 1894. Quoted by Mansfield: *Op. cit.* (3), p 25−26.

238. Power Sir d'A: The history of the amputation of the breast to 1904. *Liverpool med-chir J* NS 10:29–56, 1934.
239. Cooper WH: The history of the radical mastectomy. *Ann med Hist* 3:36–54, 1941. For a bibliography of the tabulated authors I refer to Cooper's paper and to the publications of Korteweg.
240. Korteweg JA: Die statistischen Resultate der Amputation des Brustkrebses. [Langenbeck's] *Arch klin Chir* 38:679–685, 1889.
241. Korteweg JA: Carcinoom en statistiek. *Nederl Tijdschr Geneesk* 39:1054–1068, 1903.
242. Rather: *Op. cit.* (51), p 195, note 143.
243. Borst M: *Die Lehre von den Geschwülsten.* 2 vols. Wiesbaden: JF Bergmann, 1902.
244. Ribbert H: *Die Entstehung des Carcinoms.* Bonn: F Cohen, 1905.
245. Dunphy JE: Changing concepts in the surgery of cancer. *New Engl J Med* 249:1, 1953. Reprinted in: *Milestones in modern surgery.* Hurwitz H, Degenshein GA, (eds). New York: Hoeber Harper, 1958, p 458–479.
246. Haagensen: *Op. cit.* (4), p 100.
247. Krumbhaar EB: Experimental cancer, an historical retrospect. *Ann med Hist* 7:132–140, 1925.
248. Petrakis NL: Historic milestones in cancer epidemiology. *Seminars in Oncology* 6:433–444, 1979.
249. Lane-Claypon JE: *A further report on cancer of the breast,* with special reference to its associated antecedent conditions. Ministry of Health Reports on public health, no 23. London, 1926. Quoted by Petrakis: *Op. cit.* (248) and – frequently – by Haagensen: *Op. cit.* (4).
250. Bloom HJG, Richardson WW, Harries EJ: Natural history of untreated breast cancer (1805–1933). Comparison of untreated and treated cases according to histological grade of malignancy. *Brit med J* i:213–221, 1962.
251. De Waard F, Baanders-van Halewijn EA, Huizinga J: The bimodal age distribution of patients with mammary carcinoma. *Cancer* 17:141–151, 1964.
252. Bloom HJG: The influence of delay on the natural history and prognosis of breast cancer. *Brit J Cancer* 19:228–262, 1965.
253. Macdonald I: The breasts. In: *Christopher's textbook of surgery.* Davis L (ed). Philadelphia: WB Saunders, 1964, p 339–338.
254. Hanau AN: Erfolgreiche experimentelle Übertragung von Carcinom. *Fortschr Med* 7:321–339, 1889.
255. Bra M: D'un champion parasite du cancer. *Presse méd* i:87–91, 1899.
256. Bashford EF, Murray JA: Carcinoma mammae in the mouse. *Lancet* i:798–803, 1907. Quoted by Wolff: *Op. cit.* (2), vol 2, p 68–69.
257. Slye M: Cancer and heredity. *Ann intern Med* 1:951–976, 1928.
258. Freund A, Kaminer G: Zur Diagnose des Karzinoms. *Wien klin Wschr* 24:1759–1764, 1911.
259. Yamagiwa K, Ichikawa K: Über die künstliche Erzeugung von Karzinom. *Verh jap path Ges* 6:169–178, 1916; 7:191–196, 1917.
260. Cook JW, Hieger I, Kennaway EL, Mayneord WV: Production of cancer by pure hydrocarbons. *Proc R Soc Lond [Biol]* 111:455–484; 485–496, 1932.
261. Bonser GM, Orr JW: The morphology of 160 tumors induced by carcinogenic hydrocarbons in the subcutaneous tissues of mice. *J Path Bact* 49:171, 1939. Quoted by Haagensen: *Op. cit.* (4), p 356.
262. Fischer-Wasels B: Quoted by Dietrich A: Marksteine der Krebsforschung, *Klin Wschr* 15:1297–1300, 1936.
263. Rous FP: A transmissible avian neoplasm (Sarcoma of the common fowl). *J exp Med* 12:595–705, 1910; 13:397–411, 1911.
264. Corner GW: *A history of the Rockefeller Institute 1901–1935.* New York: Rockefeller Inst Press, 1964, p 100–111.
265. Bittner JJ: Some possible effects of nursing on the mammary gland tumor incidence in mice. *Science* 84:162, 1936. Quoted by Haagensen: *Op. cit.* (4), p 355 and by Corner: *Op. cit.* (264), p 403.

266. Bordley III J, Harvey AM: *Two centuries of American medicine 1776–1976.* Philadelphia: WB Saunders, 1976, p 679.
267. Lathrop AEC, Loeb L: Further investigations on the origin of tumors in mice. *J Cancer Res* 1: 1–19, 1916.
268. Cori CF: The influence of ovariectomy on the spontaneous occurrence of mammary carcinomas in mice. *J exp Med* 45: 983–991, 1927.
269. Lacassagne AM: Un cancer d'origine hormonale, l'adénocarcinome mammaire de la souris. *Paris méd* i:233–240, 1935.
270. Matas R: In Discussion of WS Halsted. *Trans Am surg Ass* 16: 165–178, 1898. Quoted by Mansfield: *Op. cit.* (3), p 50.
271. Halsted WS: The results of radical operations for cure of cancer of the breast. *Ann Surg* 46: 1–19, 1907. Quoted by Wolff: *Op. cit.* (2), vol 4, p 56.
272. Westerman, CWG: Thoraxexcisie bij recidief van carcinoma mammae. *Ned Tijdschr Geneesk* 54: 1681–1690, 1910.
273. Lane-Claypon JE: *Cancer of the breast and its surgical treatment.* Ministry of Health, reports on public health and medical subjects, no 32. London: His Majesty's Stationary Office, 1924.
274. White WC: Late results of operations for carcinoma of the breast. *Ann Surg* 86: 695–701, 1927. Quoted by Mansfield: *Op. cit.* (3), p 38.
275. Korteweg JA: De operatieve behandeling van carcinoma mammae. (The operative treatment of mammary carcinoma). *Wbl Ned Tijdschr Geneesk* 24: 121–127, 1880.
276. Steinthal C: Zur Dauerheilung des Brustkrebses. *Beitr klin Chir* 47: 226, 1905. Quoted by Haagensen: *Op. cit.* (4), p 618.
277. Haagensen: *Op. cit.* (4), p 418–419.
278. De Moulin D: Historical notes on breast cancer, with emphasis on The Netherlands, II Pathophysiological concepts, diagnosis and therapy in the 18th century. *Neth J Surg* 33: 206–215, 1981.
279. Handley WS: Parasternal invasion of the thorax in breast cancer and its suppression by the use of radium tubes as an operative precaution. *Surg Gyn Obst* 45: 721–782, 1927.
280. Wangensteen OH: Discusssion to Taylor GW and Wallace RH: Carcinoma of the breast, fifty years experience at the Massachusetts General Hospital. *Ann Surg* 132: 833–843, 1950, p 839–841.
281. Sheridan B, Fleming J, Atkinson L, Scott G: The effects of delay in treatment on survival rates in carcinoma of the breast. *Med J Austr* i:262–267, 1971.
282. Gocht H: Therapeutische Verwendung der Röntgenstrahlen. *Fortschr Gebiete Röntgenstr* 1:14–22, 1897.
283. Körbler J: *Strahlen, Heilmittel und Gefahr.* Wien: H Ranner., 1977, p 39.
284. Perthes GC: Über den Einfluss der Röntgenstrahlen auf epitheliale Gewebe, insbesondere auf das Carcinom. *Langenbecks Arch klin Chir* 71: 955–1000, 1903.
285. Grigg ERN: *The trail of the invisible light.* Springfield (IL): CC Thomas, 1965, p 832.
286. Van der Werff JT: *De ontwikkeling der radiotherapie* (The development of radiotherapy). Nijmegen: Private print, 1965.
287. Monod R: Cancer du sein rendu opérable par la radiothérapie. Guérison se maintenant depuis trois ans et trois mois. *Bull Mém Soc nat Chir* 54: 92–94, 1927.
288. Korteweg JA: *Algemeene heelkunde* (General surgery). Haarlem: F Bohn, 1916[4]. p 534.
289. Perthes GC: Erfolge der Brustkrebsbehandlung vor und nach Einführung der prophylaktischen Roentgenbestrahlung der operierten Fälle. *Zentralbl Chir* 47: 25, 1920. Quoted by Mansfield: *Op. cit.* (3), p 73.
290. Harrington SW: Carcinoma of breast-surgical treatment and results. *J Am med Ass* 92: 280, 1929. Quoted by Mansfield: *Op. cit.* (3), p 74–75.
291. Pfahler GE, Parry DL: Roentgen therapy in carcinoma of the breast. *Ann Surg* 93:412, 1931. Quoted by Mansfield: *Op. cit.* (3), p 75.
292. Pfahler GE: Results of radiation therapy in 1,022 private cases of carcinoma of the breast from 1902 to 1928. *Am J Roentg* 27: 497, 1932. Quoted by Mansfield *Op. cit.* (3), p 75.
293. Stone: Quoted by König: *Op. cit.* (294).

118

294. König F: Betrachtungen über die Behandlung des Brustkrebses. *Zschr Geburtsh Gynäk* 87: 270–277, 1924.

295. Keynes GL: The radium treatment of carcinoma of the breast. *Brit J Surg* 19: 415–480, 1932.

296. Van Dongen JA: *Geschiedenis van het Nederlands Kanker Instituut Het Antoni van Leeuwenhoekhuis* (History of The Netherlands Cancer Institute The Antoni van Leeuwenhoekhouse). Amsterdam: Ned Kanker Inst, 1979.

297. Baclesse, F, Ennuyer A, Cheguillaume J: Est-on autorisé à pratiquer une tumorectomie simple suivie de radiothérapie en cas de tumeur mammaire? *J Radiol Electrol* 41: 137, 1960. Quoted by Mansfield: *Op. cit.* (3), p 57.

298. McWhirter R: Value of simple mastectomy in treatment of cancer of breast. *Brit J Radiol* 21: 599–610, 1948.

299. Baclesse F: Five year results in 431 breast cancers treated solely by roentgenrays. *Ann Surg* 161: 103–104, 1965.

300. Schinzinger A: Quoted by Trendelenburg F: *Die ersten 25 Jahre der Deutschen Gesellschaft für Chirurgie.* Berlin: J Springer, 1923, p 254.

301. Beatson GT: On the treatment of inoperable cases of carcinoma of the mamma: suggestions for a new method of treatment, with illustrative cases. *Lancet* ii: 104–107; 162–165, 1896.

302. Beatson GT: The treatment of cancer of the breast by oophorectomy and thyroid extract. *Brit med J* ii: 1145–1148, 1901.

303. MacMahon CE, Cahil JL: The evolution of the concept of the use of surgical castration in the palliation of breast cancer in premenopausal females. *Ann Surg* 184: 713–716, 1976.

304. Huggins C, Doa TLY: Adrenalectomy and oophorectomy in the treatment of advanced carcinoma of the breast. *JAMA* 151: 1388–1394, 1953.

305. Luft R, Olivecrona H: Hypophysectomy in man. *J Neurosurg* 10: 301–316, 1953.

306. Ulrich P: Testosterone (hormone mâle) et son rôle possible dans le traitement de certains cancers du sein. *Internat Union against Cancer* 4: 377, 1939. Quoted by Haagensen: *Op. cit.* (4), p 756.

307. Haddow A, Watkinson JM, Patterson E: Influence of synthetic oestrogens upon advanced malignant disease. *Brit med J* ii: 393–398, 1944.

308. Henderson C, Canellos GP: Cancer of the breast. The past decade. *New Engl J Med* 302: 17–30, 78–90, 1980.

309. Hagnell O: The premorbid personality of persons who develop cancer in a total population investigated in 1947 and 1957. *Ann N Y Acad Sci* 125: 846–855, 1966.

310. Gallager HS, Martin JE, Moore DL, Paulus DD: The detection and diagnosis of early occult and minimal breast cancer. *Curr Probl Cancer* 3: 846–855, 1966.

311. Zwaveling A: Bevolkingsonderzoek op mammacarcinoom. *Nederl Tijdschr Geneesk* 126: 1191–1192, 1982.

312. Virchow R: Statement made during the Kongress deutscher Naturförscher und Ärzte. Düsseldorf. 1896.

Index of names

Abulcasis 13, 14
Ackerknecht, EH 53
Aetius 3, 4, 17
Agatha, Saint 12
Aguillon, Mme d' 46
Alibert, JL 54
Alliot, JB 23, 30
Alliot, P 26
Alpinus, P 20
Anaximander 1,2
Anaximenes 1
Arceo, F 19
Archigenes 4, 5, 17
Arnott, N 57
Asklepios 2, 11, 12
Astruc, J 34, 35, 36, 43
Augustine, Saint 12
Avicenna 13

Bacalossi, P 97
Baclesse, F 102
Bailar, JC 75
Banks, M 84
Bartholin, Th 21
Bashford, EF 92
Bayle, CL 77
Beatson, GT 102–103
Béclard, PA 58
Béclère, A 99
Bell, B 45
Bennet, JH 64
Bergmann, E von 84
Bichat, MFX 37, 57, 58, 68
Bidloo, G 29
Biett, LTh 54
Billroth, Th 72–77, 81, 82, 84, 85

Birkett, J 72, 73, 75
Bittner, JJ 93
Bloom, HJG 90, 91
Boerhaave, H 32, 34, 35, 36, 37
Bonser, GM 93
Borst, M 88
Boyer, A 53, 54, 55, 62, 106
Bra, M 92
Brisbane, J 43
Broca, P 71
Brodie, B 53
Broussais, FJV 51
Brown, J (1819–62) 52
Brown, J (1735–88) 53
Bruno da Longoburgo 14, 15, 19
Burney, F 53, 55–56

Cahill, JL 103
Camper, P 32, 37, 38, 42, 44, 45, 47, 49, 97
Cancellos, GP 105
Cayol, JB 77
Celsus, AC 4, 9, 49
Cheselden, W 31, 44
Churchill, JF 77, 78, 89
Cohnheim, J 69
Constantinus Africanus 16
Cook, JW 93
Cooper, AP 70
Cooper, WH 85
Cori, CF 94
Corput, BE van den 78
Cosmas, Saint 12
Croissant de Garengot, RJ 45
Crosse, JG 54
Cruveilhier, J 51, 58, 70

Also available by the same author:

A History of Surgery
With Emphasis on the Netherlands

By **Dr. D. De Moulin**, Institute for the History of Medicine, Catholic University, Nijmegen, The Netherlands.

After a career as an active surgeon, the author of this volume switched to medical history and became Professor of the History of Medicine at the Catholic University, Nijmegen, The Netherlands.

A History of Surgery consists of original research into the development of surgery through the ages and provides a chronological survey of the events which have led to the modern achievements in surgery.
Furthermore, the book contains many historical illustrations not previously published.
There is an emphasis on surgical practice within the Netherlands. Dutch surgery, however, has by no means been taken as an isolated phenomenon: it is considered in its context within European Surgery as a whole, whilst contemporary medical thinking is set against a cultural and political background.
As a result of this unique approach, this volume will be of great interest to practicing surgeons and physicians, as well as to medical historians and the public at large.

Hardbound, 432 pp.   ISBN 0–89838–968–2
1988 KLUWER ACADEMIC PUBLISHERS

This is no chauvinistic or narrowly national history. In the compass of its 400 pages, it provides a lovely review of the history of surgery, in which an emphasis on the development of surgery and those who contributed to it is combined with a humanistic, social, and historical approach uncommon in histories of surgery. The book is necessarily brief in every section, yet the author's skill is such that the treatment of each phase is satisfyingly unhurried ... The illustrations are well chosen ... Two splendid chapters, "The beginning of Modern Surgery" and "Surgery in the Past 75 years", provide fine accounts of specific developments of surgery in the Western world during the 19th and 20th centuries. Obviously, a single chapter on 20th-century surgery can only hit the high points. The author's intention was to present a 'survey of the earlier events which led to these modern achievements ... for practicing surgeons and interns'.
He has succeeded very well.

Mark M. Ravitch, M.D.
Montefiore Hospital
Pittsburgh, PA, U.S.A.

Review in: New England J. of Medicine,
September 1988